❧❧❧ *Anita Guyton's*
# Anti-Wrinkle Plan

*By the same author:*

The Natural Beauty Book
Ageless Beauty The Natural Way

*Anita Guyton's*

# Anti-Wrinkle Plan

*How to have smoother,
more youthful skin
in just 30 days*

Thorsons
*An Imprint of* HarperCollins*Publishers*

Thorsons
An Imprint of HarperCollins*Publishers*
77–85 Fulham Palace Road,
Hammersmith, London W6 8JB

Published by Thorsons 1994


© Anita Guyton 1994

Anita Guyton asserts the moral right to
be identified as the author of this work



ISBN 0 7225 2847 7

# Contents

## Part Three: Vital Steps to Younger Skin

## Part Four: The 30 Day Anti-Wrinkle Plan

## Part Five: Some More Recipes

# Preface

None of us relish the idea of growing older, least of all *looking* old. In fact, many actually dread it. We cannot stop the passage of time but we can decelerate the deterioration that accompanies it. Smooth, unlined skin is not a matter of chronological age, money or genetic inheritance – although the latter certainly plays a part. A youthful complexion depends on

- lifestyle
- sound nutrition, high in free radicals and antioxidant nutrients
- protection against degeneration of the skin hastened by dehydration, pollutants, metabolic sludge, ultraviolet light and so on
- a state of physical and mental well-being.

It sounds straightforward enough, doesn't it, and so it is. So, why do relatively few women achieve it?

Misconception about the ageing process and ignorance about the body – including the skin and its needs for optimum health and vitality – are to blame. My aim with the Anti-Wrinkle Plan is to dispel the myth that wrinkles and the other signs of ageing are inevitable, and show that facial youthspan – like lifespan – is in your hands.

# Acknowledgements

Many colleagues have contributed to the production of this book. Unfortunately, it is impossible to thank all those involved, but I am particularly grateful to Jane Graham-Maw, Editorial Director, for her friendship, encouragement and constructive criticism, Kate Davey, her secretary, for her patience and kindness, Rosemary Staheyeff, Editor, who edited the text and had the unenviable task of condensing the index, and Lucy Daubeny and Megan Slyfield (Publicity) whose endeavours are invaluable and whose cheerfulness and optimism are uplifting.

I would also like to thank my parents, and Frederick Pridgeon and Cheryl Bernstein for all the love, support and tolerance they have shown during the last year. Finally, a big thank you to Ninian in heaven, whose love, help and encouragement prompted me to write my first and subsequent books.

To all these wonderful people, I dedicate this book.

*Part One*

# Skin and Ageing

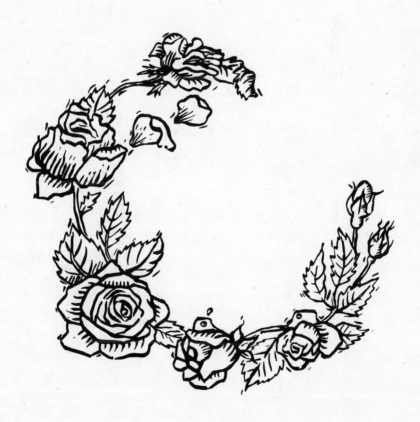

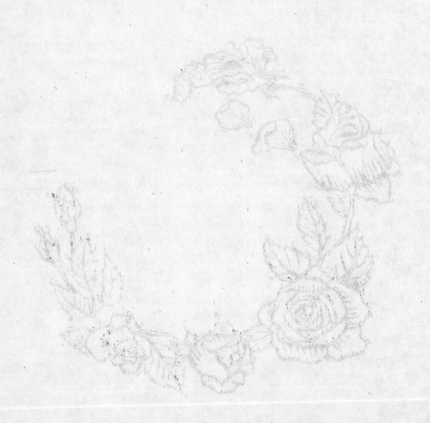

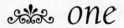 *one*

# The Skin and Ageing

## The Merciless Onslaught of Wrinkles

Wrinkles reflect the deterioration that is mistakenly called ageing. These changes begin in our early twenties and become progressively apparent as damage increases. The face communicates a wide range of emotions, from happiness to anger, and accompanying them are the laughter and the scowl lines and the frowns all of which become etched on the face. The first to appear are usually the frown lines across the forehead. Other fine lines also develop in areas where there is greatest movement and these become more marked when the skin's moisture level decreases and the neck and the cheek areas become dry.

In our thirties, expression lines deepen and those fine 'laughter lines' that fan outwards from the corners of the eyes develop into 'crow's feet'. By our forties, the fresh, smooth look of our teens has been replaced by dull, coarse, dry skin resulting from dehydration of the horny layer and atrophy of the dermis. As tissue elasticity declines, face and neck muscles lose their firmness and begin to sag. As the years slip by, more wrinkles appear on the lower and upper eyelids, making them look crinkled, and the two laughter lines running downwards from the sides of the nose to the corners of the mouth become more pronounced.

Unsightly, vertical lines appear at the base of the neck and along the upper lip, producing a puckered effect causing lipstick to 'bleed'. This is particularly common among smokers. Wrinkles continue to develop in the fifties and, to make matters worse, two prominent lines develop up the line of the platysma muscle, a muscle which extends from below the collar bone to the angle of the jaw. By now, the complexion looks pale, parched and somewhat malnourished. Before another decade of decline has passed, by which time many women have given up trying to fight what is considered inevitable, wrinkles are no longer lines but folds, and more lines progress outwards from the edges of the lips like a corrugation, produced by the muscle which closes the lips.

Additional changes also dramatically alter our appearance. During our forties, the eyes in particular are prone to puffiness below the lower eyelids, due to fat deposits and a certain amount of fluid retention. It is very common among heavy drinkers. Later however, the process appears to reverse, when fat is actually lost from the orbit, the bony cavity containing the eyeball, producing a sunken, hollow look. Further degeneration brings a creasing and a general wrinkling of the skin not only on the face but all over the body and, aided by gravity, folds of skin hang loosely – like a turkey's wattle, a noticeable example being the dreaded double or even treble chin.

# How Wrinkles Are Formed

To understand the causes of these radical changes, we must delve below the surface of the skin to the epidermis itself. Although many changes that signify old age result from maltreatment of one kind or another, certain inherent alterations do occur with time. For example, the epidermis becomes progressively thinner, making the skin look almost transparent in its fineness, but other changes are also taking place. The reproduction of cells by division, which hitherto produced perfect replicas of themselves, seems to go awry and production itself also slows down from the age of 50 onwards. It could be partly the result of genetic programming, but the major factors are damage by free radicals, oxygen molecules and the cross-linking of collagen caused by exposure to ultraviolet light, pollutants in the atmosphere, chemicals, drugs, cigarettes, alcohol, coffee and metabolic wastes. Even after sustaining damage, cells still have the ability to repair themselves to some extent, but not to the former perfection. Consequently, the resulting cells are flawed and so cellular vitality and efficiency declines and the skin begins to show signs of age.

Beneath the epidermis is the dermis, which is composed of elastic tissues known as collagen. These give skin its resilience and firmness. The thickness of the skin, which is measured in terms of the dermis, increases up to the age of 20 or so and remains fairly constant for the next 20 years before the process goes into reverse. Generally, from about 40 onwards, the dermis looks and feels thinner and veins appear where there was no evidence of them before. As a rule, the dermis is thicker in men than in women, which may account for men's skin appearing to deteriorate more slowly than women's.

As time passes, the collagen and the elastin within the dermis undergo radical changes that adversely affect our appearance. First, chains of collagen and elastin – called fibroblasts and collectively known as connective tissue – chemically bond together in a phenonenon known as cross-linking. The spirals of collagen fibres harden and bunch up to withstand this chemical attack and although this process may *seem* something of a bonus, unfortunately this is not the case. Only while these chains are smooth and resilient are they capable of absorbing moisture and snapping back into place, so plumping out the dermis and the wrinkles with it. When this cross-linking and knitting together occurs, the foundation collapses and, with no structure for the elastin to pull on, the dermis sags and wrinkles. This process is brought about by exposure to the sun, a deficiency of certain vitamins, minerals and trace elements, stress, exposure to smoke and other pollutants. Genetic programming also plays a part but to what extent is still not fully understood.

Second, the elastin fibres become unevenly distributed and ragged and not only the quality but the quantity of elastin in the dermis decreases. These changes are more evident in people between the ages of 50 and 70 than those of between 30 and 60 provided, of course, that the younger group have not been exposed to high or prolonged levels of ultraviolet radiation. Blood vessels within the dermis become smaller and so blood flow is reduced, aggravated still further by inactivity, and skin colour and poor circulation occurs. Cells deprived of essential nutrients and clogged with waste hasten malnutrition and decline on a cellular level.

Changes occur in the stratum corneum – the horny layer of dead cells on the surface of the epidermis. As new cells are formed at the base of the epidermis, existing cells push outwards and upwards towards the surface of the skin. During this process they die and dry out. Once at the surface, cells are constantly being sloughed off and replaced by newer ones from below.
Replacement of this layer occurs throughout life, but slows down significantly as the production rate of fresh cells in the epidermis decreases. During the process of ageing, both the number and the shape of the cells undergo a transformation, becoming flatter because they take longer to reach the skin's surface. This, in turn, brings about changes in the appearance of the skin. Dead cells in a young skin lie flat, smooth and close together, enabling the skin to refract light, making it smooth, soft and dewy-looking, but in older skins, the edges of the cells curve upwards, giving it a dry,

14

coarse appearance that lacks the glow that is the 'bloom of youth'. The condition and the overall appearance of the skin worsens still further when the production of sebum from the sebaceous glands diminishes, making the surface more and more dry.

Another factor that is unconnected with wrinkles and loss of elasticity, but nevertheless one which concerns many older women is the appearance of unsightly brown pigmentations, popularly known as 'liver spots' but in medical parlance called 'senile' or more appropriately 'solar' lentigines because of their association with ultraviolet light. Their appearance is due to a decline in the number of melanocytes. These are the cells that produce the tanning pigment known as melanin, which helps to protect the skin from ultraviolet damage. Melanocytes can decline by as much as 20 per cent every 10 years, particularly after the age of 30 and with this decrease in numbers comes these brown blemishes.

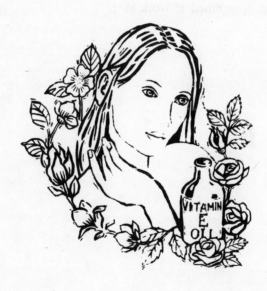

# What You Can Do

Of course, you can't avoid the inevitable if it really is inevitable. Certain fundamental changes will occur sooner or later, but because ageing, to a large extent, is deterioration either caused or accelerated by maltreatment, much of it is preventable. However, there are no magic formulas, no short cuts.

The Anti-Wrinkle Plan slows down this process of degeneration by maintaining optimum health, which involves sound nutrition, exercise, stress control, cellular damage prevention and moisture-loss protection both internally and externally and the application of substances to help prevent and repair damage on a cellular level. The time to act is when the first line appears, but even if considerable time has elapsed since then, don't despair. Wrinkles no longer signal the passage of time. Consequently, it is never too late to improve the skin or help prevent further damage, so delaying the onset of still more lines, provided you are willing and determined to work at it.

*Part Two*

# The Cause of Wrinkles and Skin Degeneration

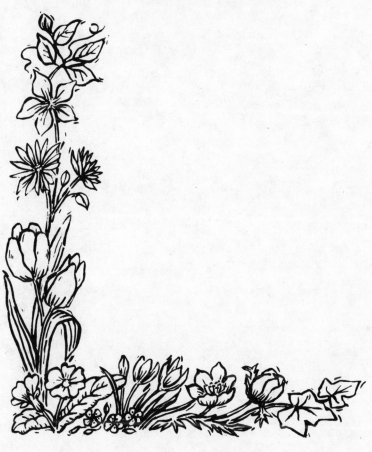

꧁ *two*

# The Causes of Wrinkles

## Overeating

Nothing deprives the face, body and mind of vitality and youthfulness more than overeating, particularly when the foods consumed are overcooked, highly refined, 'convenience' foods complete with white flour, sugar, artificial colourants, preservatives, saccharin and other chemical additives. Research has shown that women who look younger than their years consume fewer calories and that their diet is low in fat, high in fresh, raw fruits and vegetables with substantially higher amounts of vitamins A, $B_1$ and C than older-looking women of the same age.

Eating in excess of the body's needs (particularly animal proteins such as those in meat) increases the production of complex by-products, formed during the metabolization of such proteins and deposited in the tissues. This in turn encourages the formation of free-radicals which attack the cells and are a prime factor in the formation of wrinkles and other signs indicative of a collapse in cellular structure.

Reducing the calories we consume by eliminating what can only be described as 'dead' foods and replacing them with unrefined, wholefoods high in antioxidant nutrients such as vitamins A, C, many of the B vitamins and the minerals zinc and selenium and other nutrients, will dramatically check the rate at which the skin ages. It is now realized that antioxidant nutrients, both natural and artificial, if present in adequate amounts, interact to provide an on-going neutralization of free radicals. In short, they combat the damaging effects that inevitably lead to ageing.

The theory that eating less slows the ageing process, prevents age-related diseases and increases lifespan may sound far-fetched to those who believe that full stomachs fuel life, but this concept is not new. Reducing food consumption and significantly increasing its nutritional content is based on the following principles:

- all foods must be whole and unrefined: not the denatured products of refining and processing
- all foods must be as fresh as possible and preferably grown on composted, unfertilized soil. The only way to be absolutely sure that they are organically cultivated is to grow your own
- the majority of fruits and vegetables must be eaten raw to ensure that the maximum nutrients are retained
- foods for cooking should be prepared immediately prior to use and only subjected to low heat and the minimum of water. Overcooking and browning destroys the nutritional content, makes proteins difficult to digest and increases the carcinogenic (cancer-producing) properties of foods
- foods must be free of synthetic ingredients (such as colourants, preservatives and additives) not found naturally in unrefined foods
- eat small quantities of a wide selection of unrefined foods to ensure a diversity of nutrients
- eating should stop immediately hunger is satisfied – eating until you feel 'full' is eating more than you need
- use foods to nourish your body not your emotions.

My food consumption rarely exceeds 1200 calories a day, although it can be as low as 800 calories on days that are spent sitting writing.

The advantages of intermittent fasting are discussed in detail on page 68.

# Vitamin A Deficiency

Known by its chemical name of retinol and called the 'beautiful skin' vitamin, vitamin A is involved in the body's repair, protection and growth processes. An antioxidant and free radical destroyer, it protects the skin from damage and, in doing so, helps to maintain dewy, silky and young-looking skin. It is also an important antistress vitamin, an undersupply of which can lead to a vitamin C deficiency, so interfering with the maintenance and the production of healthy collagen. Other skin functions it performs include regulating the size of the sebaceous glands and preventing and curing infections – a lack of which can result in enlarged pores, acne and other infections.

In recent years, retinoic acid (vitamin A) and its derivatives have been the object of intense interest at the University of Pennsylvania where, in laboratory experiments, it was found to stimulate the growth of fibroblasts – the cells which produce new growth in the dermis and the epidermis, so speeding up the skin's natural process of repair. In addition to the production of new collagen and elastin, there was also a significant increase in the actual number of fibroblasts that were bounding with energy. These initial findings sound very promising indeed, but there is a long way to go before it is fully understood and perhaps even formulated to a preparation that can be used externally to maintain youthful skin.

What is known about vitamin A is that an undersupply, either resulting from inadequate diet or poor assimilation causes millions of cells in the lower layers of the skin to die prematurely and accumulate. This accumulation plugs pores, and prevents oil from reaching the surface, resulting in dry, scaly and rough skin. Unless corrected, this excessive dryness leads to crêpiness and early wrinkles. The skin's pores, plugged with dead cells resemble whiteheads (often mistakenly referred to as such) and they may become infected. Other common symptoms of vitamin A deficiency are dry hair that lacks lustre and sheen and is prone to dandruff, nails that peel easily and are ridged, and impaired vision in the dark, generally referred to as 'night blindness'. These disorders can be prevented and corrected by improving the diet and including foods rich in vitamin A and carotene, a substance found in yellow and green fruits and vegetables that changes into vitamin A in the body. Good sources include liver, fish and fish liver oils, eggs, whole milk, cream, butter, carrots and spinach. Also available are a wide range of vitamin A supplements.

By adding vitamin A supplements to the diet, dry skin disappears and the lubricating oils that have been missing return within weeks, although in some cases it can take longer. There is a certain reluctance to exceed the Recommended Daily Adult Dose (RDA) of 5000 IU considered necessary to maintain health because of concern about the potential toxicity of this fat-soluble vitamin. Reports of adults taking megadoses of between 100 000 and 500 000 IU daily in multivitamin and other supplement forms for a year and more have proved toxic, but these harmful effects can be prevented and counteracted by increasing one's vitamin C intake. Such high doses are unnecessary, and a waste of money, for research shows that the body is unable to use more than 50 000 IU daily. A smaller adult dose of 25 000 IU once a day or 25 000 IU twice a day for short periods under medical supervision have overcome serious deficiencies and cleared up infections, even fairly serious ones, quickly without any ill effects.

Like all nutrients, the amount of vitamin A needed by healthy people varies with each individual. Dosage must be in proportion to body-weight and so adults require more than children and men usually more than women, but the requirements of one individual with the same body-weight as another can still vary two- or three-fold according to health, age, absorption, vitamin E intake (this nutrient increases the effectiveness of vitamin A), climate, season and so on. Consequently, recommendations are of little practical use except as rough guidelines.

Longevists and age researchers using this antioxidant to slow down the process associated with ageing, take between 15 000 and 35 000 IU daily in supplement form, but never exceed this dose. If you suspect you may need to take vitamin A supplements it is best to get advice from a nutritionist, particularly if you are planning to have a baby or are already pregnant.

Vitamin supplements are part of my healthy life-style and I can't understand people who deride them out of hand. In the case of vitamin A, apart from a multivitamin and mineral tablet, which supplies 5000 IU daily, I get all I need and very cheaply too, by eating 4oz (100g) of lamb's liver 3 times a week. It provides me with approximately 83 000 IU of vitamin A 3 times a week, an average 35 000 IU daily, together with other vitamins, minerals and trace elements essential for smooth, line-free skin and optimum health.

## Vitamin B₂ (Riboflavin) Deficiency

Essential to the breakdown of all foods, vitamin B$_2$ (riboflavin) is important in many body processes, particularly tissue maintenance and the transport of oxygen to the skin's cells. Unless cellular oxygen is adequate, vital nutrients cannot be utilized efficiently or cellular wastes removed. An undersupply of this vitamin leads to malnourished, clogged cells that, in turn, lower cell vitality and hasten degeneration of the skin.

Like all the B vitamins, riboflavin is water-soluble and cannot be stored in the body. Neither is it retained in foods cooked in water, though it is fairly stable when subjected to heat. The riboflavin content is diminished still further by bicarbonate of soda and other alkalis used in cooking. However, the most drastic loss occurs when milk is exposed to light. A staggering 50 per cent of riboflavin is lost within 2 hours of exposure to bright sunlight compared with 20 per cent in dull light. Milk sold in transparent containers under fluorescent light is unlikely to contain much riboflavin if any at all.

I drink an average of two pints of milk a day, some of which is fortified with powdered milk and other nutrients, but those who don't, and that must include a large percentage of the population,

23

are almost certainly likely to be deficient in this vitamin. Indeed, research indicates that a riboflavin deficiency is one of the most widespread deficiencies in the West. A lack of riboflavin is frequently responsible for a variety of symptoms, some of which are associated quite erroneously with ageing.

Changes in the lips, resulting from a deficiency, occur quite early. Tiny, perpendicular wrinkles may be visible and lips lose their smoothness, crinkle and become rough and flake easily. As the deficiency worsens, the corners of the mouth crack (a painful condition known as stomatitis). They may heal up only to reoccur time and again. As the deficiency persists, crinkled lines of the type that appear when the mouth is puckered in a pronounced pout or a whistle become evident even when the mouth is relaxed and these may extend half-way up towards the nose. For women who take pride in their appearance, this is made worse by 'bleeding' lipstick which seeps into the lines, producing a blotchy outline. When the deficiency is only slight, the lines I have described may not appear, but lips full in youth, become progressively thinner and I have known many cases where the upper lip has disappeared almost completely. This feature is common among the elderly, but signs may appear long before one reaches middle age. The skin of people whose diets are only mildly deficient in riboflavin take on an oily appearance on the forehead, nose and chin and tiny fatty deposits like 'blind' whiteheads, appear under the skin. Abnormally florid cheeks consisting of a network of tiny blood vessels may extend from the cheeks down to the lower jaw and over the nose. Known as 'acne rosacea', this condition, which is common among alcoholics, may disappear completely when the diet is improved and vitamin $B_2$ in a B complex formula is taken with each meal, but much depends on the dosage, the degree of absorption and the severity of the condition. Other symptoms include a sore, magenta tongue, eyes that are sensitive to light and seborrheic dermatitis, a red, itchy skin condition that can spread from the head to the face, chest and other parts of the body. In contrast, extremely dry skin can also result from a lack of any one of the B vitamins and/or vitamins A and C (see pages 21, 25).

As with all vitamins, the need for vitamin B$_2$ varies with the individual. Riboflavin dosage is related to the degree of activity, so athletes and other extremely active people with well-developed muscles need more than less active people. The Recommended Daily Adult Dose (RDA) is 1.6 mg in Great Britain and 1.7 mg in the USA. However, longevitists and others suggest that the requirement is considerably higher. Consequently, to maintain optimum health to the point where ageing is retarded, a daily dosage of between 6 and 300 mg has been recommended. Decelerating the ageing process by means of dietary supplements is widely accepted. Nevertheless, bear in mind that megadoses of one or a few vitamins should never be taken unless the body is also being supplied with a good construction of all vitamins, minerals and trace elements to create a balanced interaction, enabling all nutrients to be utilized to the full.

I take 4 mg of riboflavin in a B complex or desiccated liver supplement daily in addition to many riboflavin-rich foods, such as liver and other offal, which are the richest, natural sources, yeast and steamed, leafy vegetables. With an average of two pints of milk a day, my total intake is in the region of 10 mg daily.

## Vitamin C Deficiency

A vitamin that is essential to life and health and one I am never without is vitamin C. The best natural sources of this vitamin and the bioflavonoids – substances present in foods containing vitamin C that enhance its action – are fresh citrus fruits and raw, green vegetables. However, even when daily intakes are substantial, the concentration falls dramatically during periods of stress (see page 48), leaving us susceptible to infections, fatigue, age degeneration and the symptoms generally associated with a C deficiency.

In addition to maintaining health, this water-soluble vitamin plays a vital role in the formation and maintenance of healthy collagen fibre (the protein of which healthy skin is made) and the tiny capillaries that nourish the skin cells. When vitamin C intake is inadequate, the collagen fibres in the dermis, which give skin its smoothness and elasticity, are damaged. In due course, they harden, twist and bond together in a process called cross-linking (see page 39) resulting in sagging and wrinkling skin. Also weakened by a lack of vitamin C, the capillaries break down, seeping blood into the tissues. Thus, deprived of essential oxygen and nutrients, the skin cells degenerate still further.

Another characteristic of vitamin C is its antioxidant properties. This means that it acts to detoxify radiation, industrial pollutants and other harmful substances in the body, including acetaldehyde, a toxic agent found in heavy cigarette smokers and drinkers whose consumption of alcohol exceeds the level recommended (see page 44). Without adequate vitamin C, cross-linking results. Unfortunately, many such factors responsible for skin degeneration tend to be overshadowed by dryness problems in many anti-wrinkle skin care programmes.

Vitamin C expert and author of *The Healing Factor*, Irwin Stone, and twice Nobel Prize winner Linus Pauling are among many eminent researchers who claim that vitamin C in massive doses can not only delay wrinkling and other visible signs of ageing, but is actually capable of extending maximum lifespan by as much as 35 years.

Nevertheless, the recommended daily adult dose (RDA) is still 30 mg in Great Britain and 70 mg in the USA. If Linus Pauling and other researchers are to be believed, the average person probably needs between 1000 and 5000 mg (1–5g) daily to remain in peak condition. The dosage for optimum health and age retardation can only be surmised, but evidence indicates that it could be between 10 000 and 15 000 mg (10–15 g) per day, although some experts on the subject of ageing take nearer 30 000 mg (30 g) per day.

Of course, vitamin requirements vary tremendously from one individual to the next. Age, gender, metabolism, general health, habits, climate and environment are some of the determining factors. For example, smokers lose 25 mg of vitamin C per cigarette, which means that a 20-a-day person needs 500 mg of vitamin C a day *in addition* to that needed for other bodily requirements. Daily intake needs to be increased considerably if you smoke, or drink alcohol or coffee in appreciable quantities, are under stress of any kind, take aspirin or any drugs, prescribed or otherwise, or use sweeteners or any 'foreign' substance that results in the destruction and the excretion of vitamin C.

## Vitamin E Deficiency

Vitamin E, also known by its chemical name, tocopherol, is a very versatile vitamin that has been dubbed the heart vitamin because of its reparative powers on blood clots, certain heart disorders and high blood pressure, the wonder vitamin, the antisterility vitamin, following experiments on animals, and even the sex vitamin because of its role in the production of normal sex hormones. Some claims have been the subject of much controversy, but it is its reputation as the anti-ageing vitamin and its ability to delay wrinkles and the degenerative signs associated with ageing that is of particular interest to us here. However, before assessing the virtues of this fat-soluble vitamin, let us first reconsider the primary factors that are responsible for the process that results in wrinkles, muscle wastage and pigmentation changes characteristic of old age.

Skin degeneration is the result of random destruction of the individual cells for which a number of factors are responsible. Free radicals that are the result of radiation, atmospheric pollutants and other chemicals and a by-product of the way the body utilizes oxygen, disrupt the genetic blueprint – DNA and the genetic messages – RNA – within the nucleus of every skin cell, so distorting and impairing their function and reproduction. An important side-effect of free radical attack is the phenomenon known as cross-linkage of molecules, which bond together to form a much larger structure. Locked together and unable to function correctly or to be broken down by body enzymes, these cross-linked molecules increase, resulting in a clogging and general paralysis of the cells that leads to further cellular destruction.

Vitamin E plays a vital role in actually halting this degenerative process. With its antioxidant properties, it defends the body by absorbing free radicals and the by-products of lipid (fat) peroxides in the breakdown of polyunsaturated fats, so neutralizing their destructive ability.

This antioxidant nutrient also protects vitamins B and C from oxidation and destruction and ensures a more efficient utilization of oxygen by the cells. With insufficient vitamin E to defend the cells against attack, ageing on a cellular level increases unchecked.

Dr A. L. Tappel, biochemist at the University of California and an eminent researcher and writer on vitamin E, states that the metabolic changes that occur within the cells that were once considered an inevitable part of ageing may, in many cases, be the result of a vitamin E deficiency. Furthermore, he believes that vitamin E can actually reverse the ageing process.

A brief mention has been made of the damage caused by lipid peroxides in the breakdown of polyunsaturated fats and many of you, urged on by nutritionists and beauty writers are, no doubt, including more polyunsaturated fats in your diet for the sake of healthy, line-free skin, but for the right types of oils see page 72. However, evidence suggests that people who take polyunsaturates in large doses without sufficient antioxidants such as vitamins E and C with them, develop crow's feet, wrinkles, frown lines and loss of elasticity much earlier than those who don't. I am not suggesting that oils should be excluded from the diet – far from it – but, when taking them, always make sure that you *also* include adequate vitamins E or C or both to neutralize harmful free radicals triggered by the fats. A good way of doing this is to include cold-pressed oils, which are good sources of fats and many nutrients including vitamin E. However, to be on the safe side, I boost these natural antioxidants still further by taking vitamin E (300 IU) and/or vitamin C (500 mg) at the same time.

28

By dealing effectively with the causes of skin damage, much of the ageing process can be slowed down with vitamin E.

This fat-soluble vitamin is composed of seven substances grouped under the name of mixed tocopherols, of which alpha-tocopherol is the most active in the body (so check the label before you buy vitamin E supplements). It occurs in nuts, seeds, cold-pressed oils and wholegrain breads and cereals, but the richest source is fresh wheatgerm. Certainly, natural vitamins in foods, in most instances, are preferable to synthetic, chemically produced ones, but the problem of relying solely on *foods* rich in E, is that air, heating, freezing and storing deplete the vitamin E content. Iron and iron salts destroy this vitamin within the body, but this can be avoided by taking E capsules 12 hours before or after any multivitamin and mineral tablet or any supplement containing this mineral. The best way of ensuring an adequate intake is to supplement the diet with vitamin E capsules containing 'd' or 'l' alpha-tocopherols which are biologically active (the 'd' form has a higher activity) and thus more readily absorbed by the body.

The Recommended Daily Adult Dose (RDA) considered adequate to prevent deficiency is 15 IU for men and 12 IU for women in Great Britain and 30 IU in the USA. Naturally these guidelines do not take into account fat intakes and the degree of pollutants and so on to which we are exposed daily. A consensus of opinion among nutritionists suggests that 400 IU daily is needed to maintain a healthy immune system. Many longevitists take up to 1500 IU daily, but fatty livers and other problems can result from such high doses over a prolonged period. The eminent pioneer of vitamin E therapy, Dr Evan V Shute of the Shute Foundation of London and Ontario, has treated thousands of patients with this vitamin and recommends 600 IU daily for men and 400 IU daily for women to help sustain youth and life. A sudden increase in dosage can cause high blood pressure, but this can be avoided by taking 100 IU to begin with and increasing it gradually to the level required over a period of several weeks. People with high blood pressure, overactive thyroids and heart disorders of any kind are not advised to take vitamin E in large doses.

Following breakfast, which includes wheatgerm, I always take vitamin E (300 IU) together with vitamin C and selenium, both of which work closely together and are readily absorbed when oil or fat is present in the digestive system.

## Dryness

A forerunner of wrinkles, dryness ages the skin more quickly than birthdays. Depleted of moisture, skin feels taut, like a mask several sizes too small (this feeling is particularly noticeable after washing) and, as dehydration continues, so more and more wrinkles appear. Demoisturization actually begins within the body itself and is exacerbated by external factors of one kind or another. First, let us consider the internal factors that lead to dryness and premature ageing.

### Internal Factors

#### Fat-Free Diet

A lack of internal lubrication is common among slimmers who diet constantly in an attempt to shed unwanted pounds. In striving to achieve model-like proportions, their most attractive asset – namely a young, unlined face – is likely to be sacrificed. These women are a sad sight with young trim figures and old, haggard faces. Diets abound in their thousands, but they all have one thing in common – none of them contain sufficient, if any, fats in the form of butter, nuts, seeds and cold-pressed vegetable oils, to keep every organ including the skin lubricated. Consequently, following a no- or low-fat diet for six months or more results in extreme dryness. With this comes scaliness and, if continued, a lack of fatty acids could result in eczema, dull and lustre-less hair, arthritis, vaginal dryness, menstrual problems and other disorders. The general belief is that fats, even the good ones mentioned above, contribute to weight gain, but scientific evidence suggests otherwise. Indeed, people eating too few fats of the right kind can actually become overweight. For when fatty acids are

30

undersupplied, the body converts sugar to fat more quickly than normal, supposedly in an attempt to produce the missing nutrients. Consequently, and as if this wasn't enough, blood sugar levels plummet producing hunger pangs, which are likely to lead to overeating and weight-gain. For the right kinds of fats, then, turn to page 72.

## Drinking with Meals

Once the diet has been improved to include foods naturally rich in fats and unrefined vegetable oils, their digestion and utilization must not be interfered with in any way. Unfortunately, drinking tea, coffee, water, wine or any water-based liquids with meals does precisely that. Drinking these liquids during or immediately after meals results in approximately 80 per cent of the dietary oils ending up in the liver, leaving only 20 per cent to lubricate the body and, finally, the skin. However, if soup or whole milk are taken instead, the figures are reversed with only 20 per cent finding its way to the liver, so enabling the remaining 20 per cent to oil the body and the skin. If drinking during meals is necessary (some find it difficult to masticate and swallow without liquid), make sure that it is whole milk. If you must have a cup of tea or coffee, and I enjoy tea as much as anyone, then have it 15 minutes *before* meals or about 3 hours *afterwards*.

## Acids in Liquids

Freshly prepared fruit juices are a mixed blessing. On the plus side, fresh orange or grapefruit juice from several fruits contain high levels of vitamin C and even people who don't otherwise like fruits find it a pleasant way to include them in their diet. In addition to vitamin C and its obvious benefits to health, the hydrochloric acid the juices contain aids the absorption of iron. The minus side of drinking fruits in liquid form is that it prevents the saliva salts from doing the job for which they are intended. This results in high levels of acid in the digestive and intestinal tracts and, on reaching the stomach, salts in the skin used to counteract overacidity are called into play and, as these reserves of salts are depleted, so the skin becomes dry. Fresh fruit juices and their advantages far outweigh the disadvantage, but even this slight problem can be minimized by actually chewing fruit juices. This suggestion may sound weird to say the least, but it isn't quite as strange as it sounds. Rolling small quantities as if chewing – not swishing it around like a mouthwash – helps to release the saliva salts so neutralizing the acidity. Far more harmful and with none of the nutritional benefits of fresh fruit juices are the acids in squashes and soft drinks, which being very strong and devoid of nutrients, must be avoided.

## Sunlight

High or prolonged exposure to ultraviolet light brings about degenerative changes within the skin that are ageing and potentially dangerous. Years can pass apparently without causing any adverse effects and then, suddenly, and without warning, the skin begins to deteriorate.

Under the microscope, skin normally consists of an orderly network of collagen and elastin fibres in the dermis, which are responsible for firmness and elasticity, but exposure to ultraviolet light over a prolonged period changes the basic structure into an abnormal and haphazard array of bunches and strands. Damage by free radicals and oxidation also takes place. Consequently, skin loses its firmness and suppleness, wrinkles appear, its ability to retain moisture decreases and dark areas of accumulated pigment appear, changes that are progressive and irreversible. More alarming still is that within the epidermis, cells are restructured and the distortion that occurs is considered a significant factor in the development of skin cancer.

Despite the damage and danger involved, people continue to flock to sunny shores and slopes for a suntan and faces continue to coarsen, harden, age and grow steadily more lined.

Ultraviolet radiation (UVR) can be divided into three wavelengths: UVA, UVB and UVC. Of these, the longer UVC waves don't really concern us – at least not at the moment – because little reaches the Earth and, when it does, it is filtered out by the ozone layer. Nevertheless, if ozone damage continues, it could be a problem in the future. Our main concerns at present are the UVA and UVB waves.

Until fairly recently, UVA was believed to cause little damage to the skin and, although not responsible for tanning, evidence now suggests that it can cause premature ageing. However, the culprit responsible primarily for irreparable damage to the skin is UVB. The latest hi-tech suntanning preparations aim to incorporate UVA and UVB filters to control the level of radiation, thus making sunbathing that much safer. These new products, advanced though they are, enable us to stay out in the sun longer and absorb far higher levels of sunlight than would otherwise be possible, thus significantly increasing rather than decreasing, the dangers.

Sunscreen creams or lotions should be used daily during the summer to slow down the rate at which wrinkles start to appear, whether or not you are on the beach or ski-slope. However, don't let a sunscreen, good as it may be, lull you into a false sense of security. Always remember that ultraviolet rays are powerful, destructive forces and the only way to ensure complete protection is to limit the skin's exposure to them.

Sunlamps can be just as harmful as natural sunlight. Certainly the dosage from a sunlamp is relatively small compared to sunlight in the height of the summer, but total exposure accumulated over a period of years, results in structural changes in the layers of the skin, though not obvious immediately, which will show sooner or later.

Sunbathing and sunlamps are not for me, but when exposure of some intensity or duration is inevitable, even though it may only be walking a mile or so, I still take additional antioxidant nutrients for added protection. Of these nutrients, para-aminobenzoic acid (PBA), one of the B vitamins, taken as part of a B complex formula, is helpful in protecting the skin from the ultraviolet rays. In fact, it is the main ingredient in the finest sunscreen products available and creams and salves containing PABA, applied to the skin, are also very effective.

Another group of nutrients are the carotenoids, colourants found naturally in yellow and green vegetables and fruits, that convert into vitamin A and deactivate free radicals, thus rendering them harmless. In addition to my normal diet supplemented with vitamins C and E during the summer, I take a total of 1000 mg of PABA daily and eat plenty of carrots, apricots, peppers and green, leafy vegetables.

## Wind

Sunlight has serious, adverse effects, but it is not the only environmental enemy of the skin. A common problem, particularly in winter is wind and the severe moisture depletion that results is further aggravated by the heat and the dry atmosphere of centrally heated rooms. Subjected to biting and blustery winds one minute and dry, overheated rooms the next, the skin's moisture content plummets. With this serious moisture depletion, skin feels dry, rough and unattractive.

Such problems can be prevented, or at least reduced significantly, by:

- avoiding such weather whenever possible
- wearing a long scarf to muffle most of your face
- using a good moisturizer

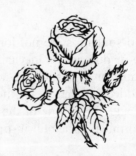

- keeping room temperatures comfortably warm but not hot during the cold months and
- maintaining humidity in the atmosphere with room humidifiers or a bowl of water in a corner of each room kept topped up.

With time the skin becomes more and more susceptible to moisture loss due to a decline in both its sebum production and water-holding ability, so give it the internal and external care it deserves. In return it will keep you looking young.

## Environmental Pollution

The sun and wind have always been with us, but air pollution is a relatively recent phenomenon. The so-called fresh air we breathe in fact is a cocktail of toxic substances – the most destructive being sulphur dioxide, carbon monoxide, nitrogen dioxide and ozone. Added to these pollutants are soot, smoke, lead from petrol fumes and other heavy metals. Air pollution is a serious problem and, unless something is done and quickly, may ultimately prove to be the major health and skin hazard of the twenty-first century.

Many toxic substances in the air also contaminate the soil. Fertilizers, pesticides and fungicides are sprayed and dusted on agricultural land annually, some of which take years to break down, thus building up to unacceptable levels in the soil. Foods cultivated commercially inevitably contain pesticide residues. Even drinking water isn't free from contaminants. In addition to the petrochemical compounds, such as insecticides, herbicides, solvents and detergents, lead and copper leached from lead and copper pipes and aluminium dissolved out of the ground by acid rain, are powerful cross-linkers found in tap water.

Individually, these substances put a tremendous strain on the body's defences, but chemicals in combination acquire heightened levels of toxicity. A good example of such interaction is fluoride, an additive in tap water and iodine. Contact with fluoride prevents the thyroid gland from utilizing the iodine and the resulting deficiency causes goitre.

Scientists believe that this myriad of substances are responsible for diseases of many kinds. Statistics show that deaths from various diseases in Britain and the USA are higher than the national average in districts where air pollution levels are greatest. Deaths from cancer and heart disease might also be linked to air pollution. In the United States, fatalities in farm animals and a number of children too were traced to nitrates from commercial fertilizers. Nitrates are also responsible for destroying or seriously diminishing the vitamin C content of crops and inducing severe liver and kidney damage in laboratory animals.

Dr Malcolm H. Hargraves, a blood specialist at the Mayo Clinic in the USA, stated that pesticides cause leukemia, Hodgkin's disease, jaundice, aplastic anaemia and other blood disorders. Extensive studies of the effects of pesticides on human health by Granville F. Knight MD and Morton S. Biskind MD reveal an alarming catalogue of symptoms, including severe depression, apprehension, anxiety and fear, fatigue and muscular weakness, shooting pains, skin sensitivity, tremors, convulsions and even paralysis. Pesticide ingestion can produce a rise in blood cholesterol, an increase in the metabolic rate, hepatitis, cirrhosis of the liver, poliomyelitis, small haemorrhages anywhere in the body, particularly the brain, heart and lungs and increase the incidence of heart disease and other conditions. Certain insecticides have produced anaemia in animals so serious that it has proved fatal. Liver and kidney damage were also evident.

The kindly face of ozone is a layer that protects us from ultraviolet radiation. However, the other side is that it is an unstable gas that, combined with other air pollutants, adversely affects the lung tissues and, as the body's inability to utilize oxygen from the atmosphere increases, so disease may occur. As if this wasn't enough, pollutants destroy the vitamin A in lung tissue needed for healthy mucous membranes, increasing susceptibility to disease.

The long-term effects on the body's organs including the skin are still not fully understood, but these oxidizing agents are believed to hasten ageing by inducing deterioration on a cellular level. What is certain is that the C, E and B complex vitamins and the mineral selenium have protective capabilities which detoxify, thus rendering harmless, pollutants and other such substances, but, in doing so, they too are destroyed.

Vitamin C is primarily known as the warrior that combats infection, but another of its roles is to remove lead, cadmium, aluminium, mercury and other heavy metals and toxic substances that come into the body by combining with them. This results in both defender and opponent being excreted in the urine, hence its use in treating chemical poisoning of industrial workers. Vitamin C also helps to protect against the potentially carcinogenic (cancer-inducing) nitrates used on agricultural land.

Vitamin E is another antioxidant that neutralizes the harmful effects of radiation from X-ray machines, ozone and nitrogen dioxide – two constituents of smog – and protects vitamin A in the lung tissues, thus increasing resistance. Riboflavin and nicotinic acid, two of the B vitamins and the mineral selenium also guard against the damage to health caused by pollution. In the USA, scientists have discovered that a diet rich in bonemeal helps to combat the fluorine accumulation in the bones of laboratory animals. Further evidence suggests that bonemeal helps safeguard against the harmful effects of radiation.

In addition to supplementing the diet with these nutrients, what other protection do we have? A diet high in natural vitamins, minerals and trace elements is of the utmost importance because, although fruits and vegetables are the vehicles for fertilizers, insecticides, pesticides and other toxic substances, these foods still contain high levels of natural nutrients necessary to neutralize harmful substances and for optimum health. The understandable but nevertheless ill-informed reasoning that a diet of overprocessed foods is the obvious way to avoid such contamination is a fallacy.

Some suggestions for protecting the skin and the body against pollution and radiation are:

- protect the skin externally by always removing pollutants from the surface of the skin with correct cleansing
- take the antioxidants C, E and B complex vitamins and the mineral selenium daily
- supplement the diet with desiccated liver, calcium, brewers' yeast, blackstrap molasses, fresh wheatgerm (vacuum packed) and cod liver oil
- improve the diet to include fresh, unprocessed foods and plenty of fruits and vegetables
- eat plenty of salad vegetables (these tend to be fairly safe and promote health)
- whenever possible, grow your own vegetables and some fruit too, even if it means planting in between flowers in a border, or buy organically grown food
- always wash fruits, vegetables and saladings well
- shell peas and peel fruits and vegetables that may have been exposed to radiation or treated with chemicals either during cultivation or afterwards to preserve them
- sprout alfalfa, fenugreek, mustard, radish and sesame seeds, aduki beans, chickpeas, lentils, mung and soya beans, sunflower seeds and wheat, rye, barley, oats and millet (they are easy to germinate in a jar and are safe and nutritionally rich sources of vitamins, minerals and trace elements)
- buy eggs from farms where DDT, BHC or chlordane are not used now nor have been in the past
- never eat in restaurants where fly sprays or aerosols of any kind are used
- don't use sprays or aerosols in the home or the garden that contain DDT, BHC, chlordane, lindane, methoxychlor or 2-4D, or better still, don't use any sprays at all.

# Free Radicals

Free radicals are an inevitable part of life, but can wreak havoc on human cells and tissues.

Free radicals are present throughout the body as a by-product of respiration. In using oxygen to provide energy by breaking down food, potentially destructive molecules called free radicals are produced that precipitate an endless process of deterioration and destruction within the body that is known as oxy-stress. It is incongruous that the oxygen-based metabolism that keeps us alive also subjects us to cellular paralysis and degeneration, a process believed to be instrumental in causing ageing.

Another source of free radical damage is the process known as lipid peroxidation. Lipids – a scientific term for fats and oils – are stored in all parts of the body as a source of potential energy and a constituent of the membrane surrounding each cell. Lipids in the body are derived from the saturated and the unsaturated fatty acids in food and are necessary to life, but unsaturated fatty acids tend to react with oxygen to form chemical compounds called peroxides, which unite with more lipids to produce still more peroxides and free radicals. This process – peroxidation – destroys the structure within and surrounding the cells and, in so doing, reduces cellular efficiency and vitality.

An important secondary effect of free radicals on cell membranes is that chemicals are formed which bond the cell's protein molecules in a process known as cross-linking (see page 26). Handcuffed in this way and unable to be released by the cells, they are prevented from performing their assigned functions. What is more, further damage is caused by congesting and choking the lysosome, a part of the cell responsible for the elimination of waste. The lysosome is an integral part of the cell and one of its duties is cellular renewal. It contains powerful enzymes capable of breaking down matter into various compartments for the purpose of rebuilding parts of the cell.

Cellular efficiency decreases with age and this results in an accumulation of partially processed 'building blocks' and insufficient material that cannot be used. Cross-linked proteins resulting from free radical attack contribute to the accumulation of unprocessed material called lipofuscin or 'age pigment' because they increase in the brain and other tissues with age, leading to age-related changes in the body.

The damage caused by free radicals and cross-linking impedes cellular nutrition, hydration, elimination and other vital functions and the loss of elasticity and firmness results in dry, sagging, wrinkled skin.

Free radical destruction also appears to be an important factor in rheumatoid arthritis – a painful and disabling disease affecting millions of people world-wide. In a healthy body, white blood cells are the so called army that defend the body from foreign organisms and part of their campaign involves discharging oxygen free radicals over the invaders. When rheumatoid arthritis strikes, the white cells advance into the joints, ejecting oxygen free radicals, which, in turn, attack the membrane of the joint, causing inflammation and swelling. The end result is the destruction of the cartilage and, ultimately, the bone itself.

To neutralize free radicals, the body has two lines of defence. First, catalase and glutathione peroxidase – two enzymes in the body – come into play. Their strategy is not direct confrontation with the free radicals but to eliminate a potential source of supply by destroying hydrogen peroxide – a form of activated oxygen which reacts with the minerals iron and copper to produce free radicals. If any free radicals escape, the second line of defence – consisting of superoxide dismutase (SOD), another anti-oxidant enzyme, and the nutrients A, C, E, beta carotene and selenium – mops them up.

In principle, this dual defence system should be sufficient to annihilate all free radicals, but external factors also trigger free radicals. These include ultraviolet rays and radiation of all kinds, air pollutants such as nitrogen dioxide, ozone and sulphur dioxide, cigarette smoke, drugs, lead, aluminium and other heavy metals. Even overeating (see page 19), is a major cause of damage by free radicals and cross-linking.

In a laboratory, with the help of a spectrophotometer to highlight, track and measure the responses of free radicals, scientists have discovered that vitamins C and E work together to neutralize free radicals – an indication that these nutrients, at least within the confines of a test tube, can prevent destruction.

Experts in free radical biochemistry, Elmer M Cranton and James P Frackelton wrote in the *Journal of Holistic Medicine* in 1984:

> The field of free radical biochemistry is as revolutionary and profound in its implications for medicine as was the germ theory and science of microbiology, which made possible development of effective treatments for infectious diseases . . . physical exercise, applied clinical nutrition and moderation of health-destroying habits all have common therapeutic mechanisms which reduce free radical destruction.

They also go on to explain the complex interaction between the body's natural defences and the antioxidant nutrients and that C and E, selenium, amino acids, riboflavin, and niacin must be present in sufficient quantities, with all the other nutrients necessary to sustain life, to interrelate and conquer free radicals, thus enabling cells and tissues to remain young and health for longer.

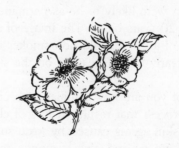

# Smoking

According to a report by the Health Education Council and the British Medical Association in 1985, smoking kills around 78 000 men and women annually in England and Wales and puts another 108 000 in hospital with cancer, heart disease, bronchitis and emphysema. The fatalities that year included my husband, who died of a coronary at the age of 63. I never really considered Ninian a smoker, for he only averaged one or two cigarettes a day, but even light smokers are at risk from coronary disease and other smoking-related disorders.

In the USA, the mortality rate is nearly three times that of Britain, with more than 300 000 deaths every year believed to be directly attributable to cigarettes. A recent survey there among 120 000 nurses revealed that those who smoke one to four cigarettes daily increase their chances of a heart attack by between two and three times. Yet, despite the mound of evidence that cigarettes endanger health and even shorten life, smoking among young women is actually on the increase.

Nicotine addicts sometimes totally disregard the health of themselves and those around them, but a fact of particular interest to women smokers is that this habit is known to accelerate the skin's ageing process. Dr Harry W Daniell, an internist in Reading, California, made an extensive study of the visible effects of smoking among 1100 patients between the ages of 30 and 70 over a 20 year period. A report of his findings in *Annals of International Medicine* states: 'Smokers in the 42 to 49 age group were likely to be as permanently wrinkled as non-smokers 20 years older'. The image of a woman of, say, 46 with the skin of a 66-year-old non-smoker is very alarming and reveals all too clearly the toll it takes on the skin.

No doubt you are now familiar with cross-linking: the degenerative process that results in loss of elasticity, wrinkles and other signs of skin ageing caused by toxic substances, especially benzopyrene, tar and carbon monoxide found in cigarettes.

42

Benzopyrene ages the skin by rapidly depleting vitamin C reserves in the body, necessary in the maintenance and rebuilding of healthy collagen. Most of us know that tar accumulates in the lungs, but few realise that it leads to a gradual build-up and release of free radicals which trigger and hasten premature ageing. Carbon monoxide harms the skin in a totally different way by binding with haemoglobin, the substance that conveys oxygen around the blood, thus literally starving the skin's cells of vital oxygen for hours at a time. All these factors combine to accelerate facial lines, wrinkles and sagging skin. However the problems don't end there. The very act of smoking, characterized by puckering the lips and squinting, which is a natural defence against smoke wafting into eyes, accentuates lip creases, particularly on the upper lip, and encourages lines around the eyes.

Even 'passive smokers' – non-smokers exposed to the tobacco smoke of others – are at risk. Carbon monoxide levels from cigarette smoke in the air can be as high as 20 to 80 parts per million, compared with the so-called safe level recommended in industrial air of only 50 parts per million. Among the lung cancers of patients who are non-smokers, 25 per cent are attributed to inhaling the cigarette smoke of others. Skin ageing resulting from exposure to this secondary smoke must be widespread and although not life threatening is still unacceptable.

Dermatologists and beauty writers who are concerned about the damage this habit is having on the skin recommend supplementing the diet with an additional 25 mg of vitamin C for every cigarette smoked daily (500 mg for a packet of 20), which is sufficient to replenish the vitamin C smoking is destroying. In my opinion, it is not only advisable but absolutely essential. Vitamin C found naturally in fruits and vegetables should also be included in the diet. In addition to vitamin C, I also recommend taking vitamin E, which helps to protect vitamin C from destruction in the body and plays an important role in cell respiration, a function that smoking impairs. It also helps prevent and counteract premature ageing.

Other preventive measures include spacing cigarettes to one or two hourly intervals, only smoking half the cigarette and using a filter, but these suggestions though helpful, are not the real solution. If you really care about ageing and want to prevent it, give up smoking altogether, hard though it may be. With all the risks involved, can you really afford not to?

# Alcohol

Like drugs or nicotine, alcohol can be addictive and extremely destructive. Taken in excess, it can damage the liver, causing hepatitis (liver inflammation) and cirrhosis, a condition in which the liver cells die and are replaced by scars, but the effects of alcohol abuse are not confined to the liver. Alcohol causes and accelerates disease throughout the body resulting in degeneration of the brain and nervous system, cancer of the mouth, throat and oesophagus, lung disease, blood disorders and increased susceptibility to infection. Heavy drinking also impedes the body's ability to absorb nutrients, a factor that leads to malnutrition sooner or later.

The majority of people who pop into a pub each day probably consider themselves moderate rather than heavy drinkers and a weekly consumption of less than 15 units of alcohol for women and 20 units for men (a glass of wine, half a pint of beer, lager or cider, one measure of spirits or a small sherry equals one unit) is unlikely to prove harmful. However, a weekly consumption that exceeds 36 units for women (the approximate equivalent of just over half a bottle of wine or 1¾ pints of beer daily) and 51 units for men (¾ bottle of wine or 2½ pints of beer daily) could jeopardize health.

A 12-year study in Hawaii showed that drinkers who consume more than half a bottle of wine a day are 3 times more likely to suffer a stroke as a result of a burst blood vessel than a teetotaller. Even abstemious drinkers who take just one glass of wine a day or the equivalent in units in beer or spirits are twice as likely to suffer a brain haemorrhage as non-drinkers.

For women drinkers, the outlook is particularly grim. Women tend to be smaller in stature and lighter in weight than men and these factors, together with a smaller liver, increase the concentration of alcohol. Consequently, women are more at risk from alcohol-related disorders than men. Furthermore alcohol is a real skin-ager. Like tobacco, alcohol causes the liver to produce acetaldehyde, a potent cross-linker that hastens ageing of the skin. Too much alcohol can also be responsible for puffy eyes and a general thinning and loss of hair. Alcohol also robs the body of the water-soluble B complex and C vitamins, causing chronic fatigue, irritability, acne, and other skin complaints, prematurely grey hair and other symptoms.

Alcohol damages the skin in other, more obvious ways. By its very nature, it is drying and this effect on the living cells leads to cellular dehydration and more and more wrinkles. The flow of proteins to the cells necessary for the maintenance and reproduction of healthy collagen is also impaired. Equally harmful is the way it inhibits the circulation of red blood cells that accumulate and obstruct tiny blood vessels, thus further depleting the cells of oxygen. The combined effects lead to damage, dehydration, starvation, suffocation and untimely death on a cellular level.

It is impossible to assess the amount of B vitamins needed daily because requirements vary with the individual and from day to day, depending on the quantity of alcohol and other liquids consumed. The dosage that is right for you is the one that makes you feel and function at your best. Admittedly, I rarely drink alcohol and therefore my B vitamin requirements are likely to be less than someone who tipples regularly. Even so, I take a small handful of brewers' yeast tablets with 500 mg of vitamin C and other nutrients immediately after breakfast and drink about 1½ pints of fortified milk, rich in protein, containing ¼ cup of powdered brewers' yeast during the afternoon. If I anticipate a long and stressful day and particularly if it is likely to include alcohol, the daily dosage is doubled to include 3 pints of fortified milk with ½ cup of brewers' yeast. Both moderate and heavy drinkers should include protein-rich foods (see page 59) in their diet to help rebuild tissues, supplemented with two B complex tablets (containing *all* the B vitamins), 500 mg of vitamin C and 2 multimineral tablets (without iron) after each meal. I would also recommend a multivitamin tablet and a vitamin E capsule containing a minimum of 100 IU of alpha tocopherol to be taken immediately after breakfast.

Finally, there is the question of calories. At approximately 50 calories for a pub measure (1/6 gill) of gin, rum, whisky or brandy, 50 calories per measure of dry sherry, Campari or Cinzano, between 65 and 75 calories for a glass of wine and about 75 calories for half a pint of beer, alcohol can't be more than an occasional treat.

# Drugs

Drugs, prescribed or otherwise, are toxic to some extent. Some drugs are more so than others. However, the toxicity in many cases is largely counteracted, though not completely, by nutrients, particularly vitamins C and E, and the mineral selenium, but the process of rendering drugs harmless prevents absorption, leading to the destruction and the excretion of these natural antioxidants. Even mildly toxic drugs interfere with the assimilation of nutrients, resulting in deficiencies that, in turn, adversely affect all parts of the body, including the skin.

Sulfonamides and antibiotics such as streptomycin and aureomycin destroy valuable bacteria necessary for the synthesis of the B vitamins, so essential to skin health. The level of vitamin C in the body needed for the maintenance of healthy collagen and the prevention of wrinkles also falls dramatically when sulfonamides, barbiturates, oestrogen, antihistamines and other drugs are taken. Tranquillizers – the crutch on which hundreds of thousands of people depend to cope with anxiety and relieve insomnia – are believed to be mainly responsible for magnesium deficiencies, a lack of which actually produces apprehension,

46

irritability, agitation, insomnia and other stress-related symptoms that the drug is meant to relieve. Prescribed drugs save lives, cure infections and alleviate suffering and, taken for short periods, are not injurious to health, particularly when the diet is more than adequate, but they can be toxic over a prolonged period.

Even those of us who don't have to take prescribed drugs of any kind are still at risk. Aspirin, a common remedy for colds and headaches, accelerates the loss of vitamins A, B and C and the minerals calcium and potassium, thus greatly increasing the need for them. Digestion and the production of tissue proteins are also interfered with, and skin deprived of these nutrients over a prolonged period, inevitably suffers. Ferrous sulphate and iron compounds, also widely available, destroy vitamins A, C, E and carotene, a substance in yellow and green fruits and vegetables that changes into vitamin A. An overdose of iron, provided it is treated quickly enough, has been counteracted by intakes of protein in large amounts and the detoxifying vitamins B, C and E.

Even a substance that is seemingly harmless like saccharin and other artificial sweeteners destroy vitamin C, causing it to be used up and excreted in the urine. In addition to artificial sweetening agents, weight-conscious women desperate to lose unwanted pounds may resort to 'water pills' in the form of diuretics, to achieve rapid weight loss, but these innocent-looking pills rid the body of water not fat and, in doing so, a potassium deficiency results. As the intake of diuretics continues, the level of potassium, which controls heartbeat and prevents dry skin, acne, dermatitis and so on drops still further, resulting in extreme fatigue to the point of exhaustion. But that is not all. With the increased flow of urine, choline, pantothenic acid, vitamin C, magnesium and all water-soluble nutrients are also excreted. The water loss from the skin cells appears as dehydration on the face and skin becomes progressively drier, which, coupled with malnutrition are responsible, in part, for premature wrinkles, loss of elasticity and signs associated with ageing.

More alarming still are the diet pills containing amphetamines that are prescribed by doctors to suppress appetite and treat depression. In addition to the considerable risk of physical and psychological dependency, amphetamines make sleep elusive and nerves jaded, so necessitating prescriptions for sleeping pills and tranquillizers. Within a short period, patients may find themselves caught in a vicious circle. Furthermore, just when nutrients are needed most and in large amounts to detoxify the drugs and rebuild health, the level actually decreases, thus undermining health still further.

Evidently the more toxic the drug, the greater the need for nutrients of all kinds. This can be achieved by generally improving the diet to include whole and unprocessed foods high in protein, and supplementing the diet with pantothenic acid (taken as part of a B complex formula) and vitamins C and E.

## Stress

Stress is part of life. It is the stimulant necessary to achievement. Contrary to popular belief, stress itself is not harmful, but the way we react to it can be. The capacity to cope with the stressors – the multiple demands and challenges that cause stress – varies from person to person. The degree of stress that is stimulating and invigorating for one person will produce tension in another, triggering migraines, irritability, insomnia, nervous fatigue, ulcers, indigestion, high blood pressure, arthritis and heart and kidney failure, to name but a few. Obviously tension that results from uncontrolled stress is extremely debilitating and a primary cause of premature ageing.

The body reacts to tension, whatever the cause, in the same way, in three, defined stages. In the first stage, known as 'alarm', adrenaline is released into the blood, which causes blood sugar and fatty acid concentrations to rise, arteries to contract, blood pressure and heart rate to increase, minerals to be drawn from the bones and these, together with other changes, mobilize in preparation for 'fight' or 'flight'.

If stress continues, the second stage is one of resistance or 'adaption' when the body is stimulated into increased activity to maintain the challenge and protect and rebuild the body with the nutrients at its disposal. If the intake of nutrients is sufficient for the body's needs, it is possible to withstand enormous stress, but immediately the reserve of nutrients is depleted and the 'exhaustion' stage is reached, illnesses and disorders develop. For example, during a day of illness or any other extreme stress, the amount of protein burned up can reach 135 g (5 oz) which is the equivalent of that supplied by 4.5 litres (8 pints) of whole milk or an incredible 37 litres (65 pints) of sterilized, skimmed milk. However, if the protein loss is replaced, the tissues remain unaffected. Unfortunately, few of us consume protein and other nutrients in quantities necessary to withstand the harmful effects of stress. As a result, the degenerative process associated with ageing accelerates.

## Nutrition

As we have seen, nutritional requirements rocket with the onset of stress. Protein intake must be increased in relation to, but not exceeding, our needs – for too much causes a mineral imbalance and, in the digestion of proteins, complex by-products are formed, which can be toxic to the system and actually hasten ageing. Therefore a nutritional balance should be maintained.

In times of great stress, the destruction of vitamin C stored in the adrenal glands is such that the need for this vitamin is increased by as much as 75 times the normal daily requirements, leaving us susceptible to colds and infections.

Another vitamin that is needed by every cell in the body to help utilize other nutrients, increase the body's ability to withstand stress, protect it against radiation damage and detoxify drugs is pantothenic acid. As with all nutrients the dosage varies with the individual and the degree of stress experienced.

Vitamins $B_2$ and $B_6$ – known as the anti-stress vitamins – are important in cellular oxidation and tissue maintenance, making them important anti-ageing nutrients.

In times of acute stress (only you can determine the degree of tension) the following supplements taken with each meal and before going to sleep are recommended. With a glass of whole milk, fortified with 2 teaspoons each of wheatgerm and powdered milk (low-fat and non-instant) take:

- 500 mg vitamin C
- 100 mg pantothenic acid
- 4 mg vitamin $B_2$
- 4 mg vitamin $B_6$.

Vitamin $B_2$ is necessary for the utilization of $B_6$ and so these two vitamins should be taken in approximately the same amounts, either in the form of brewers' yeast or a good B complex formula containing all the B vitamins.

As well as taking these anti-stress supplements three or four times daily, the diet must be complete in all nutrients, particularly vitamins A, D and E, which, in addition to protecting vitamins B and C from oxidation and destruction and the cells from damage, help rebuild new tissue, so counteracting wrinkles and muscle wastage.

When I anticipate a hard, particularly stressful day, I start the day with a generous portion of *liver* (high in protein, anti-stress vitamins, minerals and trace elements), sprinkled with wheatgerm (vitamin E) and an egg for added protein. This is preceded by two fresh oranges (for vitamins A and C). The meal ends with a glass of whole milk fortified with brewers' yeast (the B vitamins), powdered milk (low-fat and non-instant) for its high protein and calcium content, and still more wheatgerm. If stress continues, my intake of liver increases and several favourite recipes of mine using this wonderful and inexpensive food are included in The 30 Day Anti-Wrinkle Plan in Part Four.

## Relaxing stress away

Once the diet is supplemented with essential vitamins and minerals adequate to bodily requirements, one must learn to relax, for it is the only antidote to tension. Relaxation is both physically and mentally beneficial and research shows that hypertension, migraines, digestive upsets and other stress-related disorders can be alleviated or eliminated by relaxation.

One way of clearing nagging problems from the mind and restoring it to a state of inner calm is to spend part of your leisure time in recreation of a kind that you really enjoy. A vigorous walk in the woods, parkland or any green, open space restores my inner equilibrium. Other good ways are running, gardening, dancing, reading, listening to music or any pursuit that is absorbing. Furthermore, choosing a pastime involving regular exercise also helps to slow down degeneration that is characterized by poor muscle tone and sagging skin.

Many stressors are challenging but others develop out of habit and are unfulfilling, leading nowhere except to more stress. A person who was little more than an acquaintance of mine is a good example of what I mean. This person, who suffered mood swings from happiness to depression almost daily and for no apparent reason, always phoned me when he was on a 'downer', which was when I was about to serve dinner or watch a favourite programme on television; any protest on my part was totally ignored. I think he regarded me as the stimulant necessary to revive his spirits which he could tap into at any time. These phone calls, several times a week, continued for about four years. One day, I decided to eliminate all habitual stressors in my life and this was one of them. Since then, I feel and look younger, more relaxed and have far more energy than before.

If the stressor is a financial one, consider the expensive items (such as the car) and ask yourself is it a symbol of status rather than necessity and is the financial demand too great? If the answers are in the affirmative, get rid of it, at least until your financial situation improves. The tension created from the financial worry involved simply isn't worth the strain on your health and appearance.

## Relaxation technique

Total relaxation is the key that relieves the harmful effects of long-term stress, calms, reduces oxygen consumption, lowers lactate levels (high levels of which are associated with hypertension) and slows heartbeat, thus calming the mind and leaving you both physically and mentally better able to cope with life and its challenges. The simple and effective relaxation technique described here must be practised regularly for maximum benefit.

Lie on your back on a firm but comfortable floor, preferably in a darkened room. Spread your legs slightly apart and rest your arms a few inches from your body with your palms upwards. Close your eyes and take a few slow, deep breaths, inhaling and exhaling deeply. Continue this breathing pattern and, concentrating on your head, relax the muscles in your forehead, eyebrows, mouth, cheeks and jawline. When your head and face are quite relaxed, concentrate on your neck, shoulders, upper arms, working downwards to your hands and fingertips. Then, 'moving' back up your arms, relax shoulders, chest, stomach, thighs, buttocks and legs down to calves, feet, and toes. Now that your entire body is relaxed, think of yourself floating down gently into a state of deeper and deeper relaxation. Maintain this level of total relaxation for several minutes. Finally, open your eyes, stretch like a cat, and tell yourself 'now I am going to get up and feel calm and totally refreshed'.

When you practise this relaxation technique for the first time, you may not feel particularly relaxed afterwards, but don't let this discourage you. The more you practise, the deeper the level of total relaxation that will be achieved and the quicker you will be able to reach this level.

# Menopause

Although women are no longer subordinate to men and are treated as equals, when it comes to the menopause, the notion still remains that, with the loss of fertility, a woman's principal role, namely that of reproduction, is at an end. Another outmoded concept is that with the 'change of life' comes a change in attitude, a loss of value in men's eyes and with it a loss of desirability and the onset of wrinkles and old age. For women, even liberated ones, are as protective of their femininity as men are of their masculinity. These feelings of doubt and inadequacy are exacerbated by the disorders brought about as a result of changes within the body itself.

The menopause and the problems experienced differs from one individual to the next. Some women go through the change of life with little or no fuss. For others, the drop in oestrogenic (female) hormone activity manifests itself in a variety of ways. The most common changes are:

- a loss of elasticity and a decrease in hydration levels makes the skin appear scaly and dried-up and wrinkles become more pronounced
- bones become brittle and fracture easily and shrinkage in the spinal column results in a loss of height
- a decrease in hair growth under arms and around pubic area
- a reduction of fatty tissue of the pubis and the vulva.

With it comes other changes affecting the heart, the arteries, the muscles and the nervous system.

With the onset of the menopause, women may resort to hormone replacement therapy (HRT), but because of various side effects – and because HRT has induced cancer in laboratory animals – other women, like me, prefer to improve the diet and supplement it with the additional nutrients needed by the body. By so doing, many of these problems can be avoided.

During the menopause, the lack of ovarian hormones can cause severe calcium deficiency and intake of this mineral must be increased considerably if skin health is to be maintained, premature ageing avoided and demineralization of the bones averted. Calcium tablets with vitamin D to aid absorption are readily available. When the diet is good in all other respects (see page 59), irritability, depression, hot flushes, leg cramps and night sweats disappear. Calcium is also an excellent painkiller. For example, at the onset of menstruation when blood calcium levels plummet, stomach cramps can be relieved by calcium tablets taken every hour. Requirements vary from one individual to the next, but menopausal women having difficulties, and particularly anyone who cares about their skin, should take a minimum of 500 mg of calcium with vitamin D and magnesium at each meal. My average intake is 2,500 mg per day, and though not all may be needed, it is stored in the ends of the bones for future use when calcium intake is inadequate. In addition, one's intake of milk, fortified with non-instant, dried milk, should be increased.

A shrinkage of collagen that leads to wrinkles and unsightly brown blemishes commonly called 'liver spots' are evident during the change of life, when vitamin E requirements soar to new heights. These and other disorders can be averted or treated successfully with this vitamin. According to Dr N. R. Kavinoky in *Health Saver* (1959), between 10 and 25 mg of vitamin E given to 92 patients resulted in 37 of them experiencing a cessation or alleviation of hot flushes; 34 noted a reduction in heavy menstrual flow and 16 were relieved of backache. What is more, when the dosage was increased to between 50 and 100 mg it eased muscular pain and reduced high blood pressure. Night sweats also disappeared when adequate intakes of vitamin E were taken daily.

More severe menopausal disorders may be linked to stress. A good diet supplemented with nutrients to ease this condition and prevent premature ageing is required. My Stress-Reducing Menu in *Ageless Beauty The Natural Way* (Thorsons, 1993), has helped numerous women according to the piles of letters I receive, so

54

why not try it? As nerves are strained during this period of readjustment, supplementing the diet with B complex vitamins can restore calm.

Vital in protecting against wrinkles and low levels of radioactivity and in maintaining a healthy thyroid gland, iodine requirements are greatest during the menopause, when the risk of goitres, not to mention wrinkles, are greatest, but exactly how much is needed is difficult to ascertain. Unlike goitres, which are dealt with surgically, wrinkles remain, but both can be prevented by including in the diet iodinized salt, kelp, and vitamin E to ensure maximum absorption.

## Expression Lines

Expression lines are caused by frowning, scowling, grimacing, squinting, smiling, laughing or any facial response used consciously or unconsciously to express emotions or reactions in a non-verbal way become etched on our faces. Perhaps this is the reason parents berate their children for pulling faces, warning them that 'they will stay like it'. Adults, who are the worst offenders, should heed their own advice for the expressions of today become the lines of tomorrow.

I can remember that at Norman Hartnell's, the Queen's couturier, in the 1960s, there were two mannequins who were many years older than the rest, who neither laughed nor displayed any unnecessary emotion on their faces because they knew that to do so, even slightly, would give them lines. Their faces were extraordinarily beautiful but devoid of vitality.

I am not suggesting for one moment that we should do the same, but we must realize that grimaces, scowls and frowns create the sort of lines faces can do without. It will help to prevent more lines appearing although it won't minimize the lines already there. Nevertheless, lines can be softened by keeping the principal facial muscles, of which there are no fewer than 17, supple by following the 'Anti-Wrinkle Plan' and practising the facial exercises on page 82.

You may not notice these 'character' lines yourself but others will, so ask a close friend or a member of the family to point them out to you. Once you are aware of them, you can begin to control them. Alternatively, you can try this facial expression test alone at home. For this test you need a roll of transparent adhesive or hair setting tape. Place strips over the wrinkled areas of your face – along the horizontal forehead lines, the scowl lines between the eyebrows, the squint lines below the eyes and the pout lines around the mouth. Laughter lines are best ignored, for they are a small penalty to pay for happiness – a state of mind that will benefit your health, skin and keep you looking young. As you go about your daily chores (for goodness sake don't answer the door or you will look like an accident case), you will feel the tape tighten on different parts of your face. Note where it pulls and make a mental note not to make these expressions again. Control will take time but it will save a lot of unnecessary and unwelcome lines in the future.

*Part Three*

# Vital Steps to Younger Skin

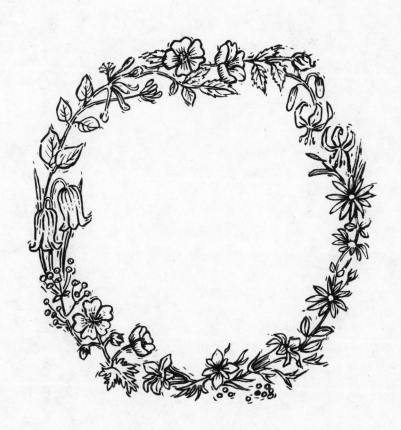

*ॐॐ* *three*

# Working From The Inside Out

## Diet

Nutrition that is high in vitamins, minerals and trace elements, using small quantities of high-quality foods without undernourishment or over-consumption is the aim of The Anti-Wrinkle Plan. The foods we eat today will form the foundation of what we are tomorrow.

Unfortunately, the foods we eat, in the main, are becoming more and more highly processed. Even those that are prepared in the kitchen from fresh ingredients are often subjected to heat so extreme during cooking that many natural nutrients are destroyed. The most popular foods are high in animal proteins, carbohydrates, salt and saturated, polyunsaturated and hydrogenated fats and low in raw fruits and vegetables, complete vegetable proteins (brewer's yeast, nuts, soya beans, soya flour and the germ of cereals) fibre and cold-pressed oils. Of these it is the latter that maintain optimum levels of health and high levels of cellular efficiency and repair necessary to slow down wrinkling and other signs of ageing.

The average Western diet is not only inadequate in nutrients needed to decelerate this process, but is likely to actually *hasten* it. Adequate protein is vital, but high intakes of *animal* protein, particularly that in meat, results in an accumulation of amyloid deposits (a fatty substance found in the tissues of big meat-eaters) that interferes with the transportation of nutrients and oxygen and the elimination of toxic material. This 'spanner in the works' of cellular metabolism hastens their decline, leading to cross-linkage and premature ageing.

The difficulty with protein is knowing exactly how much is enough. This problem is a contentious one on which scientists are unable to agree. At the turn of the century, Karl von Voit and Max Rubner recommended between 120 and 160 g (4½ and 5¼ oz) of protein per adult per day. Later, experiments by Russell Chittenden indicated that a higher level of health and performance was possible on only half that formerly recommended. This opinion was wholeheartedly endorsed by biochemist Ralph Bircher, during his life-long study into nutrition and ageing, who stated that the protein intake he recommended of between 50 and 60 g (2 and 2⅛ oz) per day was probably on the high side. Dr Miron Winick, of the Institute of Human Nutrition at Columbia University School of Medicine, suggests 46 g (1⅝ oz) per day for women and 56 g (2⅛ oz) per day for men, for maximum protection against degenerative diseases and overall deterioration. Presumably this recommendation is for people in good health, for as the late Adelle Davis pointed out, during illness or when the diet has been deficient in protein for a long time, protein intake should be increased to nearer 150 g (5 oz) per day for the first month or so.

To delay wrinkles and other signs of ageing, diet should be based on the following golden rules:

- foods must be unrefined, 'whole' foods, not denatured, highly refined and processed
- foods should be organically grown or raised as 'naturally' as possible
- fruits, vegetables and saladings should be eaten at the peak of freshness, ideally within minutes of harvesting, but this is only possible with home-produced crops. Shop produce is best purchased on the day needed, to ensure maximum nutritional value
- between 60 and 70 per cent of fruits and vegetables should be eaten raw

- a salad as part of your meal should be eaten at least once a day (see pages 175–79 for some delicious recipes)
- foods intended for cooking should be cooked very slowly using a low heat and the minimum of water – never overheat, overcook, brown or burn, for it destroys the nutritional value and creates chemicals which are potentially carcinogenic (cancer-producing) and mutagenic (the ability to change gene patterns that can be passed on to future generations)
- foods should never contain colourants, preservatives and other additives not found naturally in food
- a wide variety of foods should be eaten to ensure maximum levels of nutrition.

Following these eight rules in The 30 Day Anti-Wrinkle Plan in Part Four will provide you with a diet of the highest quality to keep you healthy, young and line-free.

## Water – The Fountain of Youth

Approximately 70 per cent of total body-weight consists of water. Blood is 90 per cent liquid, bones are 22 per cent liquid and *all* cells contain water. Water also regulates body temperature, is a perfect vehicle for transporting oxygen and nutrients to the body's cells and dissolving and eliminating toxic wastes from the tissues. Consequently water is the very essence of life.

Adequate fluid is fundamental to life and health, but, a fact often ignored, is that water is also responsible for maintaining a healthy and youthful skin. Apart from nourishing and detoxifying the system, water replenishes moisture levels in the cells, giving skin a fresh, moist and smooth appearance. Too little water and skin becomes dry, wrinkled and haggard. The signs of ageing are not only the result of loss of muscle tone but dehydration on a cellular level.

The quantity of water required each day varies, but for those in sedentary occupations in temperate climates, a fluid intake of between 1.75 and 2.75 (3 and 5 pt) is considered adequate. People who are very health conscious are likely to consume the recommended 6 to 8 glasses of plain water per day. However, fluid intake does not necessarily mean water consumption. Unadulterated water, without doubt, is a vital source of moisture that should be part of our diet, but it is by no means the only source of fluid. Neither is it the most important in terms of nutritional content. Another prime supply is the foods we eat, which contain nutrients ordinary water lacks, in addition to performing the essential functions of water in the body. As you can see from the food chart opposite, the majority of foods with a particularly high water content are the ones generally eaten raw, hence one of the reasons for a diet consisting of up to 75 per cent raw fruits and vegetables.

Although liquid in this form is nutritionally superior to plain water, all water that is pure enough to drink and unadulterated (not taken in tea, coffee, cocoa and other beverages and soft and alcoholic drinks) should be consumed daily.

## What kind of water is best?

Controversy about water purity continues unabated. If you are doubtful about the quality of your tap water or simply dislike the taste, bottled water is the only alternative.

Tap and bottled water can be soft or hard depending on the presence of calcium and magnesium. These minerals are measured in terms of grains, the fewer the grains, the softer the water. For example:

- 0 – 1 grain per 4.5l (1 gallon) is soft water
- 1 – 3 grains per 4.5l (1 gallon) is medium-hard water
- 3 – 7 grains per 4.5l (1 gallon) is hard water.

Soft water lathers easily with the minimum of soap and is nice to wash in, but it is not so appealing when it comes to preserving health. Research shows that deaths from strokes and heart attacks are significantly higher in soft water areas. Low concentrations of minerals, particularly magnesium, are believed to affect the functioning of the heart and increase the risk of death when a heart attack occurs. Magnesium, a constituent of hard water, helps reduce high blood pressure, and calcium also found in hard water,

## The Water Content of Common Foods

| Food | Percentage |
| --- | --- |
| Cucumber | 96.1 |
| Marrow | 95 |
| Lettuce | 94.8 |
| Tomato | 94.1 |
| Cantaloupe | 94 |
| Celery | 93.7 |
| Radish | 93.6 |
| Asparagus | 93 |
| Spinach | 92.7 |
| Cabbage | 92.4 |
| Watermelon | 92.1 |
| Cauliflower | 91.7 |
| Broccoli | 89.7 |
| Carrot | 88.2 |
| Milk | 87 |
| Onion | 87.5 |
| Orange | 87.2 |
| Peach | 86.9 |
| Apple | 84.1 |
| Pear | 82.7 |
| Potato | 77.8 |
| Banana | 74.8 |
| Peas | 74.3 |
| Egg | 74 |
| Cottage Cheese | 74 |
| Liver | 70.9 |
| Salmon | 67.4 |
| Chicken | 67.1 |

helps prevent osteoporosis, a softening of the bones in middle-aged and older people.

Fluoridated water is also potentially hazardous to health. When fluoridated, the fluoride combines with magnesium to produce magnesium fluoride, a salt which cannot be assimilated by the body. Consequently, this produces a magnesium deficiency which causes potassium to leave the cells, thus resulting in high blood pressure and increasing the death rate from heart disease.

Lead and copper in the pipes, chlorine believed to increase the risk of bladder cancer, arsenic from insecticides, nitrates (which interfere with the transportation of oxygen to the cells) and pollutants of many other kinds, are potentially harmful and jeopardize our chances of staying young. As I mentioned before, concentrations of heavy metals and pollutants are potent cross-linkers that hasten ageing. Keep heavy metal and pollutant ingestion to a minimum by drinking pure, mineral water and detoxifying any that may be present with the antioxidant nutrients A, D, C, E and selenium in the doses recommended.

## A Quick Guide to Bottled Water

**Chiltern (England)**  This still or sparkling mineral water originating from the Toms Hill outside Tring, is low in nitrates but high in natural fluoride. Unfortunately, the taste in my opinion, is disappointing and rather bland, but it might be just your 'cup of tea'.

**Contrexéville (France)**  A still water from Contrexéville in North Eastern France, high in lithium, magnesium and calcium, which gives it diuretic properties. It has an earthy taste that takes some getting used to.

**Evian (France)**  Still, light and extremely soft best describes this water from springs at Evian-les-Bains in the French Alps. It is slightly alkaline and low in minerals with a light taste.

*Malvern*
(England)   Bottled at the pure spring found at Malvern, this still water is passed through two filters and is described as being the purest in the world, a claim that is hard to dispute.

er (France)   From carbonated springs at Vergèze in Southern France, this naturally pure and sparkling water has become something of a status symbol among the health conscious. The carbon dioxide is removed and replaced with gas at the same controlled levels.

*y* (France)   A slightly salty and mildly carbonated water from the Vichy spa. The large number of minerals it contains is reputed to have healing and regenerative qualities. Contains fluoride.

*el* (France)   A pure, natural, still water from the Vosges Mountains containing calcium, magnesium, sulphur and fluoride. A satisfying, fairly full-bodied taste that is very pleasant.

*ic* (France)   An exceptionally pure, still water from the Auvergne Mountains in central France, with a low mineral content. It has a wonderful lively quality.
NB. Always check the labels of bottled water for trace minerals and other contents.

# Raw Juices

Those of you who are gardeners know that soil needs nutrients rich in plant foods, preferably from natural sources, to produce really robust plants and beautiful flowers. Like the flower, the skin blooms too, but only when the medium – the blood – that feeds the cells is high in oxygen, enzymes, vitamins, minerals and trace elements.

Nutrients in the sort of quantities necessary for age retardation are available naturally in foods that are fresh, unprocessed, organically cultivated and, preferably, uncooked. Fruits and vegetables are a powerhouse of nature's nutrients. A diet high in fresh foods may

65

sound boring, but as The 30 Day Anti-Wrinkle Plan Menus (see Part Four) show, they can be surprisingly delicious and their high-fibre content makes them extremely filling too.

Additional nutrients in the form of fruit and vegetable juices containing the pulp and unstrained is a pleasant and easy way of ensuring a high intake of antioxidants, one of which is pectin, a fibre of sorts that detoxifies aluminium and other heavy metals in the system by binding and eliminating them from the body. These nutrients are important in remaining young, for, as mentioned earlier, heavy metals are potent cross-linkers that inhibit the functioning of cells, eventually leading to their destruction. Though devoid of certain B vitamins, fresh fruits and vegetables are high in natural antioxidant vitamins A, some Bs, ascorbic acid (vitamin C), E and minerals zinc and selenium. They are also excellent sources of phosphorus and potassium and contain calcium, iron and sodium all of which are paramount in preventing cellular ageing.

The liquids locked in the cells of fruits and vegetables have definite therapeutic value too. Liquid fruits are the cleansers of the internal system, whereas juices from vegetables grown on organic soil regenerate and rebuild the body, including skin tissue. In fact, their regenerative powers are quite amazing, as John Lust witnessed in the interesting case concerning Mr P. O. from Wisconsin, USA. As a young man of 25 he had developed a disease of the bladder that progressively worsened during the ensuing years. By the time he was 40, he suffered pain, a burning sensation, bleeding and the usual symptoms associated with bladder disorders. Drug treatment was given but with little success. A tumour, possibly cancerous, was diagnosed and surgery recommended. By the age of 50, he was so depressed that he was considering suicide. Then he read about raw juice therapy. His gums, painful from pyorrhoea, made eating difficult so the idea of drinking raw juices appealed to him. After a three-day fast during which hot, moist packs were applied to the teeth and the bladder area, he began taking fresh juices consisting of mixtures of apples, oranges, spinach, carrots, beet, celery, cucumber and parsley. Soon, he began to feel better and, reassured, he began to restrict his intake of solid foods to raw fruits and vegetables. Mild herbal laxatives were taken to relieve constipation, though I would have preferred bran, blackstrap molasses and wheatgerm combined with natural yogurt. Toxins were eliminated including through the skin. He had a jaundiced look, lost a great deal of weight and felt unwell and miserable because of the continuous elimination. However, suddenly he began to improve, his appetite returned and his weight increased. From then onwards, he continued to recover, flabby muscles became firm and the bladder and prostate troubles cleared up. It is a remarkable case history and one of thousands that are testimony to the powers juices have for healing and regeneration.

Raw juices have been used by many medical practitioners. One such man, described by Albert Schweitzer as 'one of the most eminent geniuses in medical history', was the German physician Max Gerson. He used juices and uncooked foods high in potassium to treat a wide variety of ailments, but it was his success in treating cancer for which he is best remembered. Dr Norman Walker, the original exponent of raw juice therapy, cured himself of neuritis using raw juices and foods and lived a healthy and active life until his death at the age of 107.

Conventional theories of nutrition are unable to explain the remarkable properties of raw juices that regenerate sick bodies, lessen facial lines, firm muscles and revitalize skin and hair.

In these days of 'dead', devitalized foods, raw juices are a necessary and delicious way of feeding the body and slaking the thirst. When choosing fruits and vegetables for juicing, always select the freshest, youngest produce, preferably organically cultivated. Always wash fruits and scrub vegetables thoroughly under running water to remove insecticides and so on. Apples, pears and other fruits and vegetables with soft, edible skins should be left unpeeled. When preparing them, bear in mind that the moment they are cut, their nutrient value decreases, so juices are best prepared and drunk immediately, although they can be kept in a Thermos flask with ice for several hours if necessary.

Raw juices are extremely filling (at least I find them so) and drinking between 0.9 and 1.2l (1½ and 2 pt) a day is enough for me, although anything from 0.6 to 4.5l (1 to 8 pt) a day is recommended.

The following raw fruit and vegetable juice combinations contain the anti-ageing nutrients in high quantities:

- 7 parts carrot and 5 parts apple
- 7 parts carrot, 5 parts apple and 1 part parsley and watercress combined
- 4 parts carrot and 2 parts celery
- 6 parts carrot, 4 parts celery and 1 part spinach
- 8 parts carrot, 4 parts lettuce and 3 parts cabbage
- 8 parts carrot, 3 parts cabbage and 1 part watercress.

Some of the best fruit juices in terms of nutrient value are grape, orange, mango, guava and blackcurrant.

Carrots are a rich source of vitamin A and a good basis for mixed, raw juices, but try other ingredients and experiment with different combinations. Some concoctions you'll love, others you'll loathe, but when I consider all that concentrated goodness, even the least appetizing suddenly tastes more palatable. For more information on juices and recipe suggestions, see my book *Ageless Beauty* (Thorsons).

## Detoxifying by Fasting

For skin to be really 'in the pink', cells and tissues must function efficiently. However, if they are clogged with substances foreign to the body and waste products accumulated perhaps over a period of years, impaired efficiency results, bringing with it a lowering of vitality and a general downward spiralling known as 'growing old'.

Drugs (prescribed or otherwise), preservatives, artificial sweeteners, acidifiers, colourants and thousands of different chemicals allowed in foods and drinking water are to blame. So too, is a build-up of metabolic by-products, the primary cause being protein in excess of bodily requirements. These toxins, whatever form they take, must be flushed away if the organs (the skin is the largest organ, weighing approximately 2.75kg/6 lb) is to remain in the bloom of youth.

A detoxifying programme is a way of eliminating toxic substances and cross-linked proteins, but the type of plan must be selected with care. One way is to fast. Now the word fast means different things to different people. To the majority it conjures up an image of total abstinence, where the person concerned eats nothing and drinks only water. Such water fasts and their effects have been studied and are generally considered to be extremely dangerous.

Other types of fast are less extreme, more pleasant and, above all, much safer. These include the juice fast, the raw food fast and the fresh juice fast. Nevertheless, before starting *any* detoxification programme, it is advisable to check with a doctor who has knowledge of nutrition. Unfortunately, this isn't as easy as you might think, for such professionals are rare. So, here are some guidelines for those who find themselves without medical supervision.

## The Ten Golden Rules of Fasting

- Never fast or follow any detoxifying plan if you have ulcers, diabetes, cancer, kidney or heart disease or indeed any disease.
- Only fast or detoxify the system for a total of three days maximum without medical supervision.
- Start by eating raw fruits and vegetables, organically grown, a day before the fast, to clean the digestive tract of waste matter.
- During the fast, spend the time in a leisurely and relaxed way.
- Don't work during the fasting period.
- Never drink tea, coffee, alcohol or soft drinks or any beverages other than mineral water and raw fruit and vegetable juices organically grown while fasting.
- Don't worry if you feel temporarily worse or have a headache during the fast, for it indicates that the poisons are moving and

69

circulating through the body ready to be eliminated.

- Always break a fast properly by eating raw fruits and vegetables and a light salad, always remembering to chew slowly.
- After completing the fast, watch the foods you eat, avoiding all refined, processed foods with additives, and devitalized foods low in nutrients.
- Try to grow at least some of your own fruits and vegetables, which is the only way of ensuring that they are free of chemicals.

Here are some internal cleansing plans for you to choose from. During any internal 'spring clean' you should drink as much filtered water or bottled spring water as possible.

## Stanley A. Burroughs' Master Cleanser

Stanley Burroughs is a well-known teacher of natural health and exponent of internal cleansing.

This two-day fast involves drinking the juice of half a lemon and 2 tablespoons of blackstrap molasses (unsulphured) mixed in 250ml (8 fl oz) of medium-hot water. This drink, rich in vitamins, minerals and trace elements, can be taken between 6 and 12 times daily, whenever you feel hungry. Normal eating is resumed on the third day.

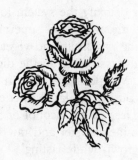

## Anita Guyton's Two-Day Cleansing Plan

This is particularly suitable for people who eat high-carbohydrate foods in large quantities.

| Day 1 | On rising | 1 tablespoon molasses (blackstrap, unsulphured) dissolved in a glass of warm spring water |
| | Mid morning | A handful of grapes (well washed) |
| | Midday | 1 glass of fruit or vegetable juice or fruit and vegetable combined (1 carrot and 1 apple liquidized is delicious) |
| | Mid afternoon | 1 cup yogurt (plain, e.g. home-made) |
| | Early evening | A small, green salad consisting of watercress, lettuce, cucumber, green pepper and raw cabbage (shredded) with a little Yogurt and Dill Dressing (see page 181) |
| | Before bed | 1 glass of spring water |
| Day 2 | On rising | 1 tablespoon molasses dissolved in a glass of warm spring water |
| | Mid morning | 1 glass of fresh fruit and/or vegetable juice |
| | Midday | 1 cup yogurt (plain) |
| | Mid afternoon | 1 piece of fruit (not citrus) |
| | Early evening | A small salad consisting of celery, cucumber, lettuce, parsley and watercress with a little Yogurt and Dill Dressing |
| | Before bed | A glass of spring water |

Note that spring water can be drunk as often as possible. This plan is intended to detoxify without causing pangs of hunger.

# Fats and Oils

Any diet, even one designed to help you lose excess weight or reduce blood cholesterol, should not be devoid of fats. The body needs fats to provide fuel, protect nerves and maintain internal organs, and utilize the fat-soluble vitamins A, D, E, and K so essential to age retardation.

Fats are broken down into fatty acids (vitamin F), many of which can be produced by the body if an undersupply occurs in the diet. The exceptions are linoleic acid, linolenic acid and arachidonic acid which are only available from the foods we eat. These essential fatty acids (EFA), so called because they are essential to life, are especially important in The Anti-Wrinkle Plan. These EFAs, found in unprocessed and unadulterated vegetable oils and nuts and seeds, maintain a moist and unlined skin by ensuring optimum levels of hydration in the skin. EFAs also halt premature ageing by ensuring that the T-cells, the fighting cells in the immune system, function efficiently. When T-cells break down or become less efficient, the immune system suffers, resulting in an increasing susceptibility to degeneration that characterizes ageing.

Fats and oils contain cholesterol, a fatty substance, high levels of which are linked to heart disease, but, as with all foods containing cholesterol, cholesterol-controlling lecithin is also present and this is an excellent source of B vitamins, choline, and inositol, which, with linoleic acid, help to lower blood cholesterol. However, there are fats and fats and you must be discriminating.

The majority of commercial vegetable oils, margarines and spreads are processed and refined to convert a natural vegetable oil, rich in nutrients, into a highly refined, clear and visually attractive product that has consumer appeal but little else. In the process of refining, valuable substances capable of reducing blood cholesterol are removed. Linoleic acid and other unsaturated fatty acids and vitamin E are destroyed. During the bleaching process, vitamin A, in the form of carotene, is lost.

Since the 1970s, the concept upheld by the medical profession was that polyunsaturated fats and oils help prevent heart disease. However, the findings of recent clinical trials have resulted in a reversal in medical opinion, particularly in the USA where recent studies show increasing incidences of malignancies in consumers of polyunsaturated products. Further findings link these over-refined products to gallstones and the sharp increase in deaths from heart disease. Perhaps most startling of all is that a drastic reduction in cholesterol levels, considered beneficial to health, may actually jeopardize it and inadvertently accelerate the ageing process. According to Dr Cedric Carne in the *Sunday Express* on 13 February 1983, a drastic reduction in cholesterol levels '. . . may lead to adverse changes in ageing cells so that they may not withstand the assault of incipient non-heart ailments'.

## Is your skin fat deficient?

The fact that you are concerned enough about wrinkles to read The Anti-Wrinkle Plan indicates that you might lack sufficient internal lubrication, which is so essential to unlined skin. Classic symptoms of a fat deficiency are dry skin and loss of tissue structure, which may be prone to acne or eczema, dull hair that is brittle with a tendency to dandruff and/or excessive hair loss, brittle nails, and frequent colds that are difficult to shake off. A fat deficiency cannot be corrected by consuming the 'bad' fats, such as fried foods, margarine, cream, animal fats, all of which, though high in fats, are low or totally devoid of the essential fatty acids necessary for health and age retardation. The 'good' fats come from unrefined, cold-pressed vegetable oils. Read the labels carefully and, if they don't say 'virgin', 'crude', 'unrefined', 'cold-pressed' or 'dehydrogenated', they are not, so don't buy them.

To avoid rancidity, all unrefined oils should be purchased in small quantities and kept refrigerated, away from light and used reasonably quickly for sautées, salads and as a substitute for saturated, polyunsaturated and hydrogenated oils and fats. When cooking, conserve the nutritional content of both the oils and the foods as much as possible. The best way to do this is to use a very low heat after 'sealing' the meat etc. to prevent loss of juices using higher but not sizzling hot heat for a short period.

## The Linoleic Acid Content in Cold-Pressed Oils

- safflower, up to 80 per cent
- sunflower, up to 68 per cent
- walnut, up to 68 per cent
- cottonseed, up to 54 per cent
- corn, up to 53 per cent
- soya bean, up to 53 per cent
- wheatgerm, up to 50 per cent
- sesame, up to 42 per cent
- peanut, up to 35 per cent
- linseed, up to 20 per cent
- olive, up to 10 per cent.

## The Approximate Linoleic Acid Content of 100 g (¼ lb) of Seeds, Nuts and Beans

- sunflower seeds, 47 g (about 1⅜ oz)
- walnuts (English, raw), 40 g (1½ oz)
- sesame seeds (dry), 20 g (¾ oz)
- Brazils (unsalted), 17 g (about ½ oz)
- peanuts (roasted), 14 g (about ½ oz)
- pecans (raw), 13 g (about ⅜ oz)
- hazelnuts or filberts (raw), 13 g (about ⅜ oz)
- almonds (dried or roasted), 11 g (about ¼ oz)
- soya beans (steamed), 3.5 g (about 1/16 oz)
- cashews (unsalted), 3 g (about 1/16 oz)

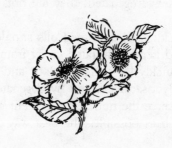

74

## Butter

Butter (unsalted), used sparingly, is best for spreading on bread and toast. Despite general opinion and for the reasons outlined earlier, margarine should not be used. Unlike margarine, butter is a wholesome, natural food, rich in vitamin A with D and E in smaller amounts. Summer butter, made from unpasteurized cream, produced while cows graze on summer pastures, contains substantially higher quantities of vitamin A than winter butter. Furthermore, it has a vitamin known as the 'Wulzen' factor that prevents arthritic-like diseases in animals.

For spreading, I combine the vitamin A content and delicious flavour of fresh butter with the essential fatty acids and their benefits into a golden spread that I have nicknamed 'mock butter'. To make it, pour 300 ml (10 fl oz) of fresh butter warmed to room temperature and 300 ml (10 fl oz) of vegetable oil (cold-pressed consisting of one or a mixture of several oils), in a liquidizer and blend until smooth. Pour the mixture into a shallow container and refrigerate. I use safflower, sunflower and sesame oils in equal parts though mixtures of other oils high in fatty acids are also good. The resultant blend is somewhat thinner in consistency than butter with a slightly nutty flavour that I find delicious.

## Cod-liver Oil

If the late Adelle Davis' opinion is correct, namely that nothing produces such beautiful children as old-fashioned cod-liver oil, than I must have been the loveliest of children. For throughout my childhood, I had to gulp down daily several spoonfuls of what to me was an obnoxious, foul-smelling oil with a taste to match. If I was unable to stomach it, there was another spoonful waiting to take its place. The daily ritual never varied and I dreaded it. Now I am grateful to my late grandmother for her foresight and insistence, but it was an unlikely beginning to what eventually turned into an affair of the skin, not the heart.

Despite, or perhaps because of these early memories, I didn't discover cod-liver oil and its virtues until many years later and quite by chance when, on medical advice, I began taking it in milk each evening. My dislike of it remained, but the pain in my back was such that it seemed the lesser of two evils. After taking the oil for several months, I noticed changes to my skin and later my hair. My skin, which was becoming increasingly dry, returned to its former moist, suppleness and, as the weeks passed, my hair took on a new lustre. Particularly important at the time was that the pain in my back gradually disappeared. I was surprised and absolutely delighted with the results, but my experience is nothing new. Cod-liver oil, with its healing and lubricating qualities, has been appreciated for centuries.

As far back as 1782, when medical knowledge was in its infancy, Dr Robert Darbey from the Manchester Infirmary wrote to a friend, 'For several years after I came to the infirmary I observed that many poor patients, who were received into the infirmary for the chronic rheumatism, after several weeks trial of a variety of remedies, were discharged with little or no relief . . . About 10 years since, an accidental circumstance discovered to us a remedy, which has been used with the greatest success, for the above complaint, but is very little known, in any county, except Lancashire; it is the cod or ling liver oil'. In those days, any disorder of the bones or joints including rickets and tuberculous joint diseases were called rheumatism.

Since then, dozens of medical reports have recorded how cod-liver oil has alleviated acne, eczema and psoriasis to anaemia, high blood pressure, emphysema, retinitis, night blindness and a host of other disorders. Then, in 1963, Dr Charles Ancoma, Director of Medicine at St Clare's Hospital, New York, submitted an article on cod-liver oil to *The Journal of the American Geriatric Society*, stating that its reducing action on cholesterol levels was greater than any vegetable oil.

Unlike the disorders mentioned above, dry, wrinkled skin is not a disease, neither is it disfiguring, painful or life-threatening,

76

otherwise more research might have been carried out on the impact of this oil as an internal lubricant and antiager. What is it about cod-liver oil that makes it effective as a healer and lubricant, particularly for the skin?

Cod-liver oil contains vitamins A and D, essential fatty acids, phosphates and iodine. As we know, vitamin A plays various roles, one of which is maintaining unlined, moist, young-looking skin (symptoms associated with a deficiency of this vital skin vitamin are considered in some detail on page 21). Known as the 'sunshine' vitamin because it is produced by the skin when exposed to the sun, vitamin D is needed for the assimilation of calcium and phosphorus, the nutrients primarily involved in bone and teeth development and maintenance and strong and healthy fingernails.

Apart from its interaction with calcium, phosphorus is needed by every cell in the body for the repair of tissues, the metabolism of sugar, the utilization of vitamins and other complex biochemical functions about which there is still much to be learned. Iodine protects against goitre, wrinkled and rough skin and the destruction caused by radioactivity. According to Carl Pfeiffer, Director of Princeton's Brain Bio Centre in the USA, iodine, along with other trace elements, may also increase longevity. As we have seen, cod-liver oil is capable of nurturing the skin in a variety of ways, but as an internal lubricant, it could be significant in keeping skin youthful and wrinkle-free.

For an in-depth assessment of your skin's moisture content, you only have to examine your ear wax (cerumen), which consists of secretions from the sebaceous and the ceruminous glands of the auditory canal. Check its colour and consistency. If the stomach is directing good-quality oil to all parts of the body, including the skin, in sufficient quantity, ear wax should be a light or a dark gold, almost amber, colour that feels soft and pasty and rather tacky. Hard and dry ear wax indicates an inadequate diet, deficient in good-quality oils. The way to improve it is to include more whole fresh foods and cod-liver and cold-pressed oils to help restore and maintain the skin's optimum moisture level and tissue structure in later years.

## How to Take Cod-liver Oil

The formula for taking cod-liver oil, which I call my 'Cod-liver Cocktail', is designed to achieve maximum lubrication of the skin throughout the body. *Note:* People with diabetes, heart disease or any disorder that makes the assimilation of oils difficult should consult their doctor.

- always take the Cod-liver Cocktail on an empty stomach, either before breakfast or, as I prefer, before going to bed, about five hours after my last meal
- to prepare, pour approximately half a cup (150 ml/5 fl oz) of whole milk into a large, empty vitamin bottle or a small jar with a screw-type lid
- if you dislike milk, use yogurt that has a fairly thin, runny consistency or, failing this, freshly prepared orange juice
- add 2 teaspoons of cod-liver oil – either the plain or the flavoured variety
- don't substitute cod-liver oil capsules, believing that the results will be the same – they won't
- shake the Cod-liver Cocktail vigorously for about 20 seconds until it is frothy
- drink immediately (if you are unable to obtain the flavoured kind and dislike the taste and the smell of the ordinary variety, hold your breath while drinking it and breathe through your mouth until you have brushed your teeth)
- after taking the Cod-liver Cocktail, don't eat anything for at least one hour
- continue to take the Cocktail for at least six months
- if, after this period, you want to either reduce or discontinue it, do so gradually by taking it every alternate date and then every third day and so on.

# Exercise

The body is a complex machine that needs 'working' regularly if it is to function efficiently. Apart from helping us to live longer, exercise can slow down and actually prevent the decline that affects the body with age. Exercise stimulates the system into action, transporting oxygen and nutrients to all parts of the body and eliminating wastes more efficiently, thus hastening repair. It increases longevity by reducing high blood pressure, controlling blood sugar levels and body weight, so lessening the risk of heart disease. By using sugar to produce energy, exercise is also proving helpful in controlling diabetes. Regular workouts may also counteract depression, increasing the production of noradrenaline, which induces feelings of euphoria and well-being. It aids age-prevention by slowing down and even reversing the onset of osteoporosis, a disease in which calcium is lost from the bones, making them brittle and liable to fracture easily.

Another degenerative process associated with ageing is the replacing of muscle with fat. Evidence suggests that the average person loses 225g (½ lb) of tissue and replaces it with 450g (1 lb) of fat annually between the ages of 35 and 65. This means that over a 30-year period, you and I are likely to lose 6.75 kg (15 lb) of valuable tissue and cloak the shrinking frame with 13.6 kg (30 lb) of fat, hence the tendency to become either scrawny or fat in old age. However, vigorous exercise tones and builds up muscle and burns up fat, thus inhibiting muscle wastage whilst restricting the accumulation of fat.

I am the first to admit that 'pumping iron' by jogging, weight-lifting or long distance running doesn't appeal to me any more than it does most people, but the fact remains that muscle tissue begins to deteriorate within just 24 hours of inactivity. Imagining the changes that take place after a year or more without exercise is enough to frighten even the worst lounge lizard into activity. Choose an aerobic exercise like brisk walking, swimming, skipping, rowing, cycling or aerobic workouts, which involve vigorous, sustained energy as opposed to squash, an anaerobic exercise requiring sudden bursts of energy that can cause high blood pressure and so increase the risk of heart attacks.

Exercise sessions of 30 to 45 minutes duration, at least 3, preferably 4 or more times a week, not only promote health but make you feel and look younger, too. Increased blood flow brings colour to the face and oxygen and nutrients to the skin's cells, while eliminating waste material that clogs the cells.

James White, an exercise physiologist at the University of California at San Diego, carried out a study on the extent to which exercise taken regularly retards and reverses skin ageing. Results showed that older women who followed a programme of regular exercise using mini-trampolines looked younger, had better skin colour and fewer wrinkles than younger women who took no regular exercise. It was also found to reduce bags under the eyes.

Exercise need not be strenuous to the point of exhaustion to do you good. The less energetic will be delighted to know that research indicates that there is an upper limit of exercise beyond which no additional benefit to the heart is evident, as well as a lower limit below which health benefits are not obvious. Exercise needs to be vigorous enough to make you out of breath but not so winded that it prevents you from talking or singing (see the Pulse Rate Guide, opposite). If tightness across the chest or any pain or discomfort in the upper body, including the throat, is experienced, stop immediately and consult your doctor.

Even if you are really fit, and few of us are, walking a total of 100 miles a week is no more beneficial to health than 20 miles per week, so there is no need to walk or jog yourself into the ground. Naturally, clocking up 20 miles a week, the upper limit, would be a struggle for anyone whose only activity is climbing out of bed in the morning, but it can be achieved if you work up to it slowly. If you are a fairly sedentary person most of the time, unfit and starting from scratch, don't throw yourself wholeheartedly into strenuous workouts. Exercise, whatever form it takes, should be at a relaxed pace to begin with and increased gradually over a period of weeks and months. Begin your programme of exercise by changing your life-style: walk instead of drive to the shops, take the stairs, not a lift, and give the dog an extra daily walk, fairly briskly round the park. Walking upstairs is an excellent form of exercise, so why not start using your own stairs to ease yourself back into shape.

Walking at a good pace and enjoying it in green, open spaces appears to be the best, natural exercise for most people. It also has the advantage of being inexpensive, needs no special equipment apart from a comfortable pair of walking shoes, is least likely to cause injury and lifts the spirits, inducing a feeling of mental well-being and inner calm. Whatever form of aerobic exercise chosen, the energy and feeling of vitality and well-being it induces encourages us to take even more.

## Pulse Rate Guide

For each exercise session to have maximum effect, the pulse rate (heartbeats per minute) should be between 70 and 75 per cent of the maximum pulse rate. Here is a guide to help you.

| Age | Maximum pulse | Exercise range | |
|-----|---------------|----------------|--|
| | | 70 per cent | 75 per cent |
| 20 | 200 | 140 | 150 |
| 25 | 195 | 136 | 146 |
| 30 | 190 | 133 | 143 |
| 35 | 185 | 129 | 138 |
| 40 | 180 | 126 | 135 |
| 45 | 175 | 122 | 130 |
| 50 | 170 | 119 | 127 |
| 55 | 165 | 115 | 123 |
| 60 | 160 | 112 | 120 |
| 65 | 155 | 108 | 115 |
| 70 | 150 | 105 | 112 |
| 75 | 145 | 101 | 108 |
| 80 | 140 | 98 | 105 |

Take your pulse at the neck or wrist after 10 minutes of continuous exercise. Use the second hand on a watch or clock to count to 10 seconds and count your heartbeat. Multiply your pulse rate by 6. Now compare it with the exercise range columns. If it is below the 70 per cent recommended, the exercise is not vigorous enough, so go a little faster, but comfortably so, in the next 10-minute session.

## Facial Exercises

Make-up improves the surface of the skin by disguising tiny flaws and imperfections, but wrinkles, bags, crow's feet, drooping eyelids (resulting from slackness, not heredity), jowliness and sagging contours are by no means superficial. These are structural changes within the very foundation of the face that occur when muscles weaken and shrink and succumb to the pull of gravity.

Years ago, women had only two alternatives. The first was to accept these changes as inevitable and resign themselves to looking old or resort to plastic surgery, which is extremely expensive and temporary. However, today's women can correct these structural weaknesses and prevent further muscle decline by exercising daily within the privacy of their own homes. In the same way that exercise can reshape and recondition flabby body muscles to become supple and firm, so exercises can do the same for the muscles in the face.

Facial exercises strengthen the muscles and, as they firm up, the skin becomes contoured and smoother. A wrinkled, sagging face is rather like an old cushion: reinforce the padding and the creases almost disappear. Exercise is the means by which a similar effect can be achieved for the face. Exercising the face also increases circulation, bringing fresh supplies of oxygenated and nutrient-rich blood to this area, thus further stimulating and toning the skin.

Such exercises are not new. For years, experiments were tried with little if any success. A number of researchers studied facial anatomy, and their findings resulted in a series of scientifically formulated exercises that really work. Now I am not promising miracles, but practised regularly and correctly as part of your daily routine, they can prevent and correct muscle deterioration, thus reducing jowliness and smoothing out sags, creases and lines that give the appearance of age.

The best time to do these exercises is early in the day when you are fresh and relaxed. Always use petroleum jelly to lubricate the areas to be exercised.

## To Strengthen Under-eye Muscles and Eliminate Lines and Bags Below the Eyes

Standing in front of a mirror, lean towards it so that your arms are resting on a shelf, table or wash-basin.

Looking at your eyes in the mirror, slowly lift the lower lids upwards, in a series of tiny movements. This is actually much more difficult than it sounds, but try it once or twice to begin with, gradually increasing to five movements upwards and five movements downwards, when your eyes will be almost closed. Repeat twice.

## To Strengthen Under-eye Muscles

In the same leaning position as above, raise your eyebrows slightly and slowly raise your lower lids in a series of tiny movements until your eyes are half closed, as if you are screwing them up against smoke.

Next, close your eyes slowly and squeeze the lids tightly together while relaxing your eyebrows. Hold tight to the count of five.

Gradually relax the squeeze and, with your eyes still closed, release the lower lid muscles in a series of five movements. Open your eyes and relax. Repeat twice.

## To Strengthen Drooping Upper Eyelids

Still in front of the mirror, support each side of the head with your thumbs. Placing your index fingers under your eyebrows and holding firmly against the bone, close your eyelids slowly. You should feel a downward pull from eyebrow to eyelid.

Squeeze your eyelids tightly together and hold to the count of five.

Relax and squeeze slowly and hold to the count of five. Relax. Repeat twice.

## To Strengthen Cheek Muscles

Still in front of the mirror, with your lips slightly apart, imagine a fine line running from the corner of your mouth to the lobe of your ear. Now, move the left-hand corner of your mouth along that imaginary line in a series of five slow movements, holding to a count of five after each movement (to a count of 25 in total).

Now, move the corner of your mouth back again in five slow movements, holding to a count of five after each movement. Relax.

Now exercise the right-hand corner of the mouth in the same way. Repeat once each side.

## To Strengthen Lip and Surrounding Muscles

Still facing the mirror, open your mouth slightly as if to say 'oh!' Now, drop your lower jaw in eight, slow movements, while slowly moving the corners of your mouth inwards. On the eighth movement, your mouth should be oval in shape and the areas around the mouth very tight.

Holding this position, place all eight fingers on your chin to hold it downwards and then stretch your top lip outwards towards your cheeks in a series of five slow movements, keeping your mouth oval in shape, and hold and count to five after each movement. (This movement can be difficult until you learn to master your muscles.)

Now, with your upper lip stretched outwards, move the lip back in five movements, pausing after each movement. Remove your fingers and relax. Repeat twice.

## To Strengthen Cheek, Neck and Mouth Corner Muscles

Still facing the mirror with your teeth and lips slightly apart, move the corners of your mouth in two slow movements, concentrating particularly on moving the lower lip: first, half-way towards the sides of the face and hold to a count of five, second, move them as far back as possible, doing so very slowly, and hold the resulting position to a count of five.

Next, slowly return to the half-way position and hold it to a count of five. Relax.

When you can do this dual-movement, two-part exercise easily, move on to the next stage.

Try to increase the number of movements from two to five. Slowly, as before, move from the first movement to the fifth movement, holding to a count of five after each movement. Relax. Repeat once.

## To Strengthen and Streamline Jawline and Eliminate Jowls

In front of the mirror, tilt your head up and push your chin forward.

Next, slip your upper lip down behind your lower teeth, gripping your upper lip with your teeth. (You'll feel your neck and jawline muscles contract.)

Now smile up and out towards your ears in five, slow movements and hold to a count of five.

Move your lips back in five, slow movements. Gradually release your lips and relax. Repeat twice.

# Treating the Outside

## Cleansing

The skin can be nourished internally and externally with nutrients and moisturizers, but unless it is 'squeaky clean', it will look neither healthy nor beautiful. Cleansing is the most important part of any skin care programme and requires three kinds of cleansers. The first is a water-in-oil cleanser (one of the greasy types) that glides on and removes all make-up and surface grime. Next comes an oil-in-water cleanser (cleansing milks belong to this group) to remove the oil and any remaining surface dirt and, finally, soap, which is a superb cleansing agent. The only valid criticism is that, being extremely alkaline, ordinary soap reduces the skin's natural acidity, leaving it open to bacterial infection, but this can be corrected by applying an acidic, non-alcoholic freshener (see page 88).

Like many women, I have tried dozens of oil-based cleansers, but unrefined vegetable oils (cold-pressed rather than heat treated to retain all the natural nutrients), though expensive compared with highly processed vegetable oils, remain the cheapest and in my opinion, the most efficient cleansers, for removing make-up, particularly waterproof mascara. Unrefined safflower, sunflower, walnut, corn, soya bean and other such oils should be purchased in small quantities and stored in the refrigerator to prevent oxidation.

To cleanse, pour a little oil onto the palm of the hand and apply it evenly over the face, working it in gently with the fingertips.

Wait for one minute (to enable it to absorb the make-up and grime accumulated during the course of the day), then remove it using a pad of moist and absorbent cotton wool. Repeat the process.

The second stage involves the removal of the oily residue and any remaining traces of make-up using cotton wool dipped in either dairy milk or conventional cleansing milk. An extremely efficient water-based cleanser, dairy milk leaves the skin really clean and vibrant-looking and differs from other cleansing milks in that it doesn't leave the skin feeling dry and taut.

The third stage is to wash the skin in warm, not hot, water using a white, non-perfumed and non-adulterated soap. Super-fatted soaps containing lanolin, 'cream' and other fatty ingredients are a good advertising ploy but nothing more. They have neither the same cleansing efficiency of unadulterated soaps nor the ability to moisturize the skin as claimed. In fact, it is impossible, if soap is to be washed off as it should be. Furthermore, if soap is to cleanse properly, it doesn't leave a film of grease or anything else for that matter, on the skin. Despite claims to the contrary, cleansing and moisturizing are two separate and diametrically opposed actions that can only be achieved separately.

When washing, we tend to use too much soap, assuming that the more lather there is, the cleaner the skin will be, but this is another misconception. Only a *little* soap – little more than a fine smear – is needed to keep the skin beautifully clean. Using only a trace of soap and your fingertips, massage it lightly all over your face, including every fold and crevice. It should be done efficiently but quickly (within about 60 seconds), to ensure maximum cleansing without adversely affecting the hydrolipidic film (see page 88), a reduction of which makes dry skin even drier. Now, rinse thoroughly 15 times with warm, not hot, water followed by cool, not cold, splashes. This cleansing routine should be carried out once a day at least, preferably at night when accumulations of dirt are highest, but not more than twice a day.

# Why we Need a Freshener

The surface of the skin is covered with a hydrolipidic film – an emulsion composed of water from the sweat glands and oil from the sebaceous glands – that acts as a natural moisturizer, and, being slightly acidic, also guards the skin from bacterial and chemical attack. This so-called 'acid mantle' is extremely important and needs to be maintained.

Unfortunately, soaps and cosmetics, most of which are rather alkaline, destroy this protective film, enabling moisture to escape more rapidly and leaving the skin more susceptible to infection. Consequently, though marvellous skin cleansers, soaps encourage dehydration and this is particularly apparent after washing when skin feels uncomfortably 'tight'. Generally, soaps in Britain do not carry the pH level on the label, which, for the sake of our skin, should be in the region of 5. However, with a strip of litmus paper (available from chemists) you can test the pH for yourself. If the paper stays a yellowish colour, the pH reading is fairly acidic, but if it turns blue, it is very alkaline and if it reaches purple, discard the soap altogether! A more general guide is that the more the soap lathers, the more alkaline it is.

The skin's natural acid mantle can be restored by applying a freshener with cotton wool immediately after washing and before moisturizing. Commercial fresheners come in three strengths according to their alcoholic content as follows:

## Fresheners

These consist of an aromatic ingredient dissolved in water with a little alcohol sufficient to soothe and tighten the pores and restore the skin's acid balance without actually drying it.

## Toners

Their higher alcohol content, which produces a slight tingling sensation, makes them suitable for normal skins.

## Astringents

These are the strongest of all, with a high percentage of alcohol, producing a temporary tightening effect on the pores that is extremely drying and only suitable for oily skins.

## A *fresher for all skin types*

Obviously older skins that are already dehydrated and wrinkled need a freshener that is capable of restoring the acid balance without drying it still further. A simple freshener that suits all skins, whatever the degree of dryness, can be made at home for a matter of pennies and is as follows:

**Acid Mantle Replacement Formula**
1½ cups (15 fl oz) of spring (bottled) water
1 teaspoon cider vinegar

Simply combine the ingredients and pour into a bottle with a screw-type lid and label. Apply with cotton wool immediately after washing and before moisturizing.

# Moisturizers

Despite what cosmetic companies say to the contrary about the relative merits of their creams to penetrate deep within the horny cells, lubricants, emollients, moisturizers, or whatever other name they go by, do not penetrate the skin to any extent. What they do is remain on the surface where the action is, as an invisible barrier to moisturize preventively by halting, through their impermeability, the process of transpiration in which moisture in the cells evaporates into the atmosphere. The principle is similar to that which keeps a chicken moist covered with cling-film. While inhibiting moisture loss, this barrier also shields the skin from pollutants and other toxic substances in the atmosphere.

Skin loses moisture and is under threat of one kind or another constantly and so a moisturizer of some kind must be used ·to protect the skin at all times. Petroleum jelly and vitamin E oil (see pages 92, 94) each have special characteristics that are essential in The Anti-Wrinkle Plan. Cold-pressed vegetable oils are also important.

My preference for home-made creams and lotions made from dairy cream, eggs, vegetable oils and other 'live' foods rich in enzymes, vitamins, minerals and trace elements to encourage moisture retention and retard skin ageing is well-known. For example, the extremely high fat content of fresh, double cream (48 per cent) makes it undesirable as a dietary food, but it is this very ingredient that, combined with its water content, makes it a superb water-in-oil emulsion for moisturizing the skin. Then there is the vitamin content to consider. One tablespoon (½ oz) of fresh, double cream contains over 200 IU of vitamin A, with vitamins D and E in smaller amounts – all of which can be absorbed and are needed in skin maintenance.

A good moisturizer, be it from the kitchen or the laboratory, must maintain moisture balance in the horny cells to prevent dehydration. It must also bind cells that curl up at the edges, a phenomenon dermatologists believe may be at the heart of moisture loss and dry skin. The stratum corneum is composed of cells that ordinarily lie flat and slightly overlap, like the scales of fish, forming a barrier against moisture loss. However, these flattened cells can curl up, leaving the way open to transpiration. The greasiness of water-in-oil moisturizers seals and smooths down the edges, leaving the skin feeling soft, moist and dewy-looking.

Commercial brands come in a wide range of formulas and textures, but the oil-in-water emulsions are the ones most widely used. Being relatively high in water and low in oil, they are light, fluffy, non-greasy and delightfully cool and pleasant to use. However, their moisturizing ability is negligible because the water content, though high, evaporates rapidly and what fat there is, is insufficient to protect the skin from drying. In fact, if they are applied regularly to normal skin over a prolonged period, they actually encourage the horny layer of the skin to dry out.

The best way to prevent and alleviate demoisturized skin is to change to a water-in-oil emulsion, called 'cold' or 'all-purpose' creams in the United Kingdom. Containing more fat than water, these moisturizers feel more greasy as a result, spread evenly over the epidermis, so encapsulating moisture and thus preventing dryness. Despite their proven efficiency, it is surprising how few are available. The ones I have found, instead of being displayed prominently on cosmetic counters, were difficult to find – I really had to search for them. Instead, space was devoted almost exclusively to the inferior oil-in-water creams. This is not surprising really considering that they are produced more cheaply, water costing far less than oil, and heavier, more frequent applications are needed, so they provide a higher level of profit.

Naturally, it is much easier to prevent dehydration and other problems that accelerate skin ageing than to hydrate and undo the damage of years. The visual evidence of skin that has become progressively demoisturized day after day and year after year, aggravated by nutritional and internal lubricant deficiencies resulting from an inadequate diet, exposure to extremes in weather conditions and the degeneration caused by free radical damage, pollution and other hazards to which skin is subjected, won't disappear in a matter of days. The Anti-Wrinkle Plan, if followed, will bring about a steady improvement and friends will begin to notice and comment on how much younger you look, but treatment must be continuous, morning and evening, day after day, year after year. Spasmodic treatment, just when you remember, won't work.

## Petroleum Jelly

Petroleum jelly, a derivative of petrol, commonly known as Vaseline, is included in many cosmetic creams, hand lotions and baby products for its moisturizing, lubricating and emollient effects, but is it really the humble ingredient we believe it to be? Evidence suggests otherwise. However, to appreciate its action, it is necessary to understand the scientific foundation on which moisturizers are based.

On the basis of I. H. Blank's experiments published in 1952, cosmetic scientists suggested that there are three methods of action by which a moisturizing agent can work. The first, called 'occlusion', is where the agent traps moisture in the skin by forming an impermeable barrier over the stratum corneum, the layer of dead cells above the epidermis. Second, the 'humectant' way is where the agent draws and binds extra water from the atmosphere to the skin. Finally, 'water delivery' is where water is incorporated in the moisturizer, so enabling additional moisture to be massaged into the skin.

For many years petroleum jelly has been regarded as the 'occlusive' moisturizer par excellence. However, if its action *is* occlusion, its benefits would disappear as soon as it was washed off. Experiments reveal that this is not the case. Petroleum jelly applied to the skin daily for one week reduces dry, scaly skin. However, what is particularly interesting is that these beneficial effects continue for a further week after treatment before skin returns to its former condition. With a three-week treatment, symptoms of dryness are eliminated completely and the skin remains not only moist but supple three weeks later. These revelations have led to speculation that petroleum jelly is capable of actually rejuvenating the outer skin, the epidermis, thus inducing more youthful characteristics in the stratum corneum. If, in fact, petroleum jelly *does* affect the epidermis, a three-week treatment would eliminate dryness in the stratum corneum for the entire three weeks of its life, which is precisely what happens. Further evidence shows that in actually penetrating the skin, petroleum jelly induces changes that lead to a gradual thickening of the epidermis, a factor that could help to counteract the natural and progressive thinning of the epidermis that occurs with the onset of age. Obviously petroleum jelly is an excellent lubricant and moisturizer for alleviating dry skin – one of the prime causes of wrinkles – but it is not by occlusion only, though by what other method(s) remains a mystery.

It goes without saying that I am never without petroleum jelly! Nevertheless, I have to admit that it is not the easiest or the most pleasant of moisturizers to use, but don't let its consistency or smell discourage you from using it. Apply it to a thoroughly clean skin, over the entire face, including the delicate skin under the eyes, and the neck, carefully, without pulling the skin. Leave for 15 minutes and then tissue off the excess. Splash the face and neck with hot water, and pat dry.

## Anti-Wrinkle and Antioxidant Skin Food
100 IU vitamin E capsule
7500 IU vitamin A capsule
½ teaspoon ascorbyl palmitate (oil-soluble vitamin C powder*)
8 drops evening primrose oil
4 drops wheatgerm oil
½ teaspoon petroleum jelly

Pierce the ends of the vitamins E and A capsules and squeeze the contents into the ascorbyl palmitate powder. Add the other oils and mix together until the paste is smooth and spreadable. Work in the petroleum jelly thoroughly. Apply the mixture liberally over the face and neck and massage in gently without pulling the skin.

When I am working at home, I apply it after washing in the morning and leave it on for the remainder of the day. On the other hand, when I have to go out, I leave it on for half an hour, preferably longer, and then tissue off the excess before applying make-up.

* Available from smaller pharmacies and by post from Nature's Best, PO Box 1, Tunbridge Wells, Kent TN2 3EQ.

**Anti-ageing Skin Food To Help Protect Against
Free Radical Damage**
4 tablespoons petroleum jelly
600 IU vitamin E capsule
2 teaspoons ascorbyl palmitate (oil-soluble vitamin C powder, see
page 93)
2 teaspoons wheatgerm oil
2 teaspoons sunflower oil
1 teaspoon evening primrose oil
1 teaspoon cod-liver oil
1 teaspoon carrot oil

Melt the petroleum jelly over a low heat. Remove it from the heat
and put it aside to cool. Meanwhile, pierce the vitamin E capsule,
squeeze the contents into the ascorbyl palmitate powder and mix
until smooth. Next, add the remaining oils and mix thoroughly
before adding it to the petroleum jelly. Continue to stir until the
mixture is smooth and spreadable.

Apply the skin food evenly and gently over the face and neck
without pulling the skin. Leave for a minimum of half an hour
before tissuing off the excess and applying make-up.

## Vitamin E Oil

Vitamin E that is taken internally in the form of foods or
supplements plays an important role in the formation and
maintenance of healthy skin tissue (see vitamin E deficiency on
page 27). Particularly interesting, however, is the action of vitamin
E oil when used topically, or directly on the skin.

Experiments into stress and premature ageing carried out by the
Austrian scientist Dr Hans Selye, Director of the Institute of
Experimental Medicine and Surgery at the University of Montreal,
show that vitamin E fed to young rats in large doses can prevent
wrinkles and other signs associated with the ageing process. If so,
then what effect if any does it have when applied directly to the
skin of humans?

This question was answered by one of the world's great authorities on nutrition, Adelle Davis, who reported that when vitamin E capsules were pierced and squeezed on to scars produced by burns, the scars disappeared. These findings were upheld by another eminent nutritionist, Dr Carlton Fredericks, during an interview on American television, who explained how vitamin E oil applied directly to skin wounds may actually retard healing, but that it does result in less noticeable scars after the healing process is completed. Recent experiments carried out by Peter T. Pugliese of the Xienta Institute of Skin Research in Bernville, Pennsylvania, also shows that, applied to the skin, vitamin E oil helps repair damaged capillaries that leech out into surrounding skin tissue, a problem that occurs increasingly with older people who live on devitalized, highly refined foods.

Linda Clark in her book *Secrets of Health and Beauty* (1969) reports excitingly on the way vitamin E oil erases lines from the skin. She carried out an experiment among a group of friends, consisting of several women, two men and herself, into the effects of vitamin E oil on the skin over a four-week period. After cleansing the skin night and morning, each member of the group punctured a 200 IU vitamin E capsule with a pin and applied the golden substance to various parts of the face. Miss Clark collected the reports from each person four weeks later and those who used the oil twice daily were enthusiastic about the results. The member(s) who applied it to lines under the eyes reported that they were less noticeable. One woman commented that her crêpey skin was tighter as a result and a third noticed that tiny lines on the upper lip had smoothed out. The sallow skin of another woman had acquired an attractive, pinkish glow and she also reported that the oil made her face feel warm. Other participants who applied their favourite moisturizer over the oil did not achieve the same noticeable results. So, it seems, vitamin E oil applied externally as well as taken internally has positive and noticeable benefits on the skin.

Curious, I decided to try an experiment of my own, the only difference being that I would use the contents of a 300 IU capsule once each evening rather than those of a 200 IU capsule twice a day. I punctured the capsule and applied the liquid to the skin under my eyes, where minute lines were beginning to form as a result of skin puckering in laughter, which, as anyone who knows me well will confirm, is something I do freely and frequently. These lines are so fine that they are barely noticeable but I realize that in time, they are likely to deepen, so this was the area on which I concentrated. Each evening, I dabbed the contents of a 300 IU capsule containing d-alpha tocopherol, the most biologically active of all, on to the skin. I didn't notice that the treated area felt warm or indeed any change in skin tone, both of which were reported by members of Linda Clark's group. In fact, I didn't notice any improvements at all. As the weeks passed, I was beginning to doubt these reports, but I continued and I am pleased that I did. On the fifty-ninth day my laughter lines had smoothed out and as the treatment progressed, so they became less and less noticeable.

## Unrefined Oils

As we know, unrefined vegetable oils, rich in essential fatty acids (EFAs), particularly linoleic acid, in the diet improve moisturization and put the brakes on cellular ageing (see page 73). However, like all nutrients, EFAs can also be absorbed through the skin's surface and application directly to the skin either from capsules or unrefined vegetable oils that contain them, ensures rapid assimilation where they are most needed. Applied in this way, they actually strengthen the hydrolipidic film, unlike many commercial moisturizers that, due to their alkalinity, destroy it. They also strengthen cell walls, resulting in a more efficient channelling of nutrients and elimination of wastes and increase the moisture retentive capacity of the skin.

Wheatgerm oil, containing approximately 50 per cent linoleic acid, is a favourite of mine which I massage into my skin daily. Another is sunflower oil (cold-pressed), an excellent source of EFAs that, applied regularly, dramatically improves the texture and the appearance of the skin. The reason my skin remains unlined when that of my contemporaries are suffering a mid-life cellular crisis is, I am sure, due to regular application of these unrefined oils.

A recipe of mine which I call Anti-Wrinkle and Antioxidant Cream (or AWAOC for short), consists of several oils high in linoleic acid and other fatty acids and antioxidant nutrients to combat damage and general wear and tear at cellular level. Why not try it?

**Anti-Wrinkle and Antioxidant Cream**
½ teaspoon ascorbyl palmitate (oil-soluble vitamin C powder, see page 93)
7 drops wheatgerm oil
7 drops sunflower oil (cold-pressed)
7 drops evening primrose oil
7500 IU capsule vitamin A
300 IU capsule vitamin E

Pour the ascorbyl palmitate powder into an egg cup. Add the oils. Pierce the ends of the vitamins A and E capsules and squeeze out the contents. Mix thoroughly with a spatula. Apply the mixture evenly over the face and neck and massage gently without pulling or dragging the skin. Skin that is really hungry will soak it up like a sponge.

# Exfoliating

Exfoliating is a mild form of skin peeling, designed to deep cleanse by gently removing the dead cells from the surface of the skin, using slightly abrasive but harmless natural or artificial substances.

This sloughing off of the dead cells which, if allowed to remain make skin rough, flaky and clog the pores, thus inhibiting normal skin activity, is an important skin care treatment, but exactly how it works is still not fully understood. The theory is that the production of epidermal cells over a period of time must equal the rate at which cells are shed. Therefore, gently removing the dead cells on the skin's surface must stimulate the epidermis below into producing more young cells.

Normally, a young skin renews its surface layer every two or three weeks whereas an older skin can take between four and six weeks. Consequently, exfoliating activates the epidermis to significantly increase cell production.

'Exercising' the skin in this way has other benefits too. The gentle friction also stimulates the flow of rich blood to the face, thus nourishing, rebuilding and regenerating the tissues. Practised regularly, it also firms the skin, which I can only attribute to the stimulation induced by the friction. Men slough off these dead surface cells while shaving each day, and this, I am convinced, is the reason older men's skin tends to look younger than their years.

Women of all ages need to exfoliate but how frequently depends on the condition of the skin. If you have dry or normal skin that is rough and looks dull, try once and twice weekly treatments respectively. For so-called 'combination' skin, treat the forehead, nose and chin areas which are oily two or three times a week and the cheeks which are dry to normal once a week. Skin that is ultra-sensitive should be treated with the gentlest exfoliator once a fortnight. Obviously, whatever your skin type, never overdo the treatment, always remember to moisturize afterwards and never go out in the sun following treatment.

Exfoliators range from complexion brushes, manually or battery operated, to synthetic sponges specifically designed for this purpose, and abrasive creams and cleansers that remove cellular debris while cleansing the skin.

If you are trying this treatment for the first time, use nothing more abrasive than a clean, slightly coarse (but not too rough) face flannel. Wet it in warm water, wring it out, drape it over one or two fingers and rub it over the surface of the skin, in every

98

fold and crease, using gentle, circular movements, for several minutes. Then, splash your face with cool water 12 times, pat dry and moisturize.

As your skin gradually grows accustomed to the treatment, change to a synthetic sponge or a soft, bristle brush. Wet your face and dab the sponge or the brush in your favourite soap or cleanser and with small, circular movements, work evenly all over the surface of your skin. Splash your face with cool water 12 times, pat dry and moisturize. Alternatively, use one of the natural ingredients below.

## Natural Exfoliators

### Oatmeal
Pour a small quantity of fine oatmeal into the palm of your hand. Add a few drops of warm water and mix to a coarse paste. Massage it gently on to clean, wet skin, using small, circular movements. Rinse with cool water, pat dry and moisturize.

### Sea salt
Pour a little fine (not coarse) sea salt into the palm of your hand and rub it lightly on to clean and slightly wet skin, but don't overdo it. Rinse with cool water, pat dry and moisturize.

Sea salt is not suitable for delicate or sensitive skins.

# Three in One Skin Care Treatment

A friend of mine had a beautiful, wrinkle-free complexion that made her look at least 20 years younger than her 74 years. Her skin was amazing and the envy of many younger women. I asked what her secret was several times, but she smiled and replied 'One day'. Years later, just before she died, she revealed the secret of that lovely, unlined skin.

Apparently, twice daily, morning and evening, after cleansing and washing, she massaged sunflower oil (unrefined) all over her damp face for a minute or so. Next, several drops of juice from a freshly squeezed lemon were applied on top of the sunflower oil and massaged in until it felt rather sticky. Then, fine sea salt was poured into the palm of her hand and worked gently all over the oily areas, including under the eyes. She finished by splashing her face 15 times with clean, hot water and patted dry, leaving an invisible and protective film of oil.

This Three in One Skin Care Treatment is invaluable in four ways. First, it lubricates and nourishes the skin with high-grade oil, rich in natural nutrients and linoleic acid, which, you may recall is important in maintaining a young, unlined complexion. Second, the lemon juice, high in vitamin C, ensures the correct acid/alkaline balance. Finally, the sea salt removes all the dead cells on the surface of the skin and in doing so, also stimulates cell production and efficiency.

# Natural Skin Tighteners and Wrinkle Erasers

### Raw Egg Formula
Cleanse, wash and pat the skin dry, then apply raw egg white over the face. Leave it on for 10 to 15 minutes. Rinse it off with tepid water followed by cool water splashes. It leaves the skin feeling clean, smooth, firm and wonderfully 'alive', but, unfortunately, the tightening effect is only temporary.

After preparing my Complexion Cocktail for Dry Skin (see page 185), I dip my fingers into the egg shell containing the white residue and smooth it all over my face. By doing so, I give my skin two beauty treatments for the price of one without taking up any extra time!

### Lecithin Formula
Dissolve lecithin granules in a little warm water and combine this mixture with safflower or sunflower oil (cold-pressed) until it is

smooth. Massage this creamy mixture into the skin for on-going care throughout the day. Rich in vitamins B and E and fatty acids, it revitalizes skin tissue but must be used regularly over a period of months.

### Honeyed Egg Formula
Blend 1 egg, 1 teaspoon of raw honey and 1 tablespoon of dried milk to a smooth and spreadable paste. Add a little whole milk if necessary. Apply to the face and leave it on for as long as possible. Remove with tepid water followed by cool water splashes. The softening, tightening and slightly astringent effect imparts a lovely glow to the skin, leaving it feeling silky and smooth.


# Facial Massage

Massage is an ancient art that revs up the circulation while relaxing the mind and the body. Facial massage can be extremely beneficial, but unfeeling and unskilled hands that work roughly and in all directions can break the connective fibres, stretching and actually damaging the skin, causing more harm than good. However, when done correctly and gently, following the direction of the facial muscles, massage improves the blood circulation responsible for transporting nutrients to the cells and flushing away cellular sludge, thus improving the tone of the muscles and the skin and imparting a healthy glow to the complexion, thereby helping to keep it firm, supple and resilient. Massage also encourages the skin to absorb active nutrients in cold-pressed oils and the home-made moisturizers mentioned earlier.

Always begin a massage by oiling the skin of your face and neck with sunflower or any other cold-pressed vegetable oil.

### Movement 1
Beginning with effleurage (meaning massaging with the flat of your hand and your fingers in a stroking motion), starting from your collar bone, run your hand up the front of your neck and under

your chin to above the jawline. Now repeat with your other hand. Repeat nine times with each hand.

## Movement 2
Again, using effleurage, in gentle strokes starting at the jawline, move them up over the cheeks, over the eyes and up the forehead to the hairline and back down again in one unbroken movement. Repeat five times.

## Movement 3
With the middle and third fingers of each hand, starting at the bridge of your nose, make a circular movement outwards along the eyebrow, round the cheekbone and back to the nose. Repeat five times.

## Movement 4
With the third finger of each hand, starting from the tip of your nose, run your fingers up your nose, out over the inside corners of your eyebrows and up your forehead to your hairline. Repeat five times.

## Movement 5
With your index fingers at the sides of your nose and your thumbs under your jawbones, curve your hands up and outwards along the cheekbones and jawbones simultaneously (so the curve gently presses the whole cheek area) to your hairline near your ears. Repeat five times.

## Movement 6
Holding the tips of your fingers as if you are playing the piano, play your ten fingers all over your face in a tapping and lifting motion.

## Finishing
Finish the massage by removing the excess oil left on your skin with a wad of cotton wool dipped in milk. Splash your face with warm water several times and pat dry. Apply a freshener with the correct acid/alkaline balance, followed by a moisturizer.

*Part Four*

# The 30 Day Anti-Wrinkle Plan

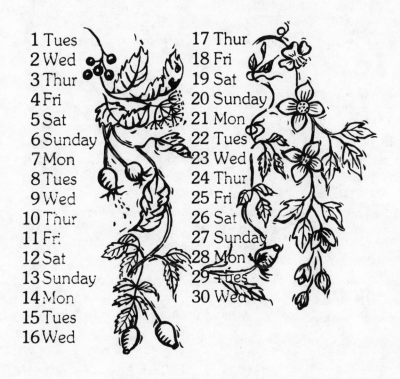

| | |
|---|---|
| 1 Tues | 17 Thur |
| 2 Wed | 18 Fri |
| 3 Thur | 19 Sat |
| 4 Fri | 20 Sunday |
| 5 Sat | 21 Mon |
| 6 Sunday | 22 Tues |
| 7 Mon | 23 Wed |
| 8 Tues | 24 Thur |
| 9 Wed | 25 Fri |
| 10 Thur | 26 Sat |
| 11 Fri | 27 Sunday |
| 12 Sat | 28 Mon |
| 13 Sunday | 29 Tues |
| 14 Mon | 30 Wed |
| 15 Tues | |
| 16 Wed | |

# ❀❀❀ *five*

# The 30 Day Anti-Wrinkle Plan

## Menus

- The lunch menus can be served at dinner and the dinner at lunch if this is more convenient.
- Alternate the breakfast cereals for variety and maximum nutrition.
- All cooked meals should be cooked as slowly as possible using a low heat.
- The cup measurements used are British cups, the equivalent of 10 fl oz.
- Refer to the table on pages 166–67 for detailed information on vitamin and mineral supplements.

## Day 1

*On Awakening*  1 or 2 glasses of water

*Breakfast*  1 or 2 oranges
Breakfast cereal with 1 tablespoon of wheatgerm
1 glass of health drink of your choice or whole milk. Vitamin and mineral supplements

*Lunch*  Piece of fresh fruit of your choice (optional)
Broad Bean Salad
1 glass of whole milk

*Dinner*  Piece of fresh fruit of your choice
Haddock à L'Orange with jacket potato (optional) and side salad of your choice
1 glass whole milk and vitamin and mineral supplements

*Before Bed*  Cod-liver Cocktail (see page 78), to be taken at least four hours after eating

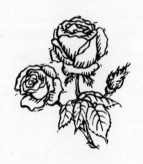

## Broad Bean Salad

*Serves 1–2*

Cook the beans until tender and leave to cool. When the beans are cool, mix the oil and the lemon juice together and pour over the cooked beans. Blend the yogurt and the cottage cheese together and pour over the beans.

*750g (1¾lb/2 cups) broad beans*
*1 teaspoon vegetable oil, cold-pressed*
*juice of ½ lemon*
*300ml (10 fl oz/1 cup) plain yogurt*
*100g (4oz/½ cup) cottage cheese*

## Haddock à L'Orange

*Serves 2*

Place the cutlets in a greased, ovenproof dish and season with freshly ground black pepper. Pour over the orange juice. Sprinkle on the grated orange rind, onion. Top with the cheese and breadcrumbs, pour over the vegetable oil and bake at a low heat until cooked. Serve with jacket potatoes and side salad of your choice.

*2 haddock cutlets*
*freshly ground black pepper to taste*
*juice and grated rind of 1 small orange*
*1 tablespoon grated onion*
*4 teaspoons grated cheese*
*4 teaspoons wholewheat breadcrumbs*
*25ml (1 fl oz) vegetable oil,*
  *cold-pressed*

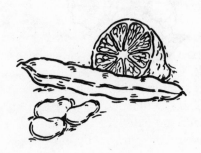

# Day 2

*On Awakening*   1 or 2 glasses of water

*Breakfast*   1 or 2 oranges
Poached or scrambled egg on 1 or 2 slices of wholemeal toast or breakfast cereal with 1 tablespoon wheatgerm
1 glass of health drink of your choice or whole milk. Vitamin and mineral supplements

*Lunch*   Piece of fresh fruit of your choice (optional)
Tuna and Red Kidney Bean Salad
1 glass of whole milk

*Dinner*   1 piece of fresh fruit of your choice
Country-style liver with sliced apple and green salad
1 glass of whole milk and vitamin and mineral supplements

*Before Bed*   Cod-liver Cocktail (see page 78)

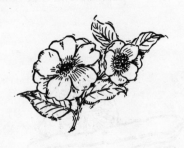

## Tuna and Red Kidney Bean Salad

1×185g (6½oz) tin of tuna, drained
1×400g (14oz) tin of red kidney
   beans, drained, or 2 cups cooked
   red kidney beans
salad dressing of your choice (see
   pages 179–81)
1 onion, sliced
1 avocado, peeled, stoned and diced
fresh chopped parsley to garnish

**Serves 2**
Toss the tuna and the kidney beans in the salad dressing, place the onion and the avocado on top and garnish with parsley. Serve with watercress, and a jacket potato (optional).

## Country-style Liver

1 medium onion, thinly sliced
1 tablespoon vegetable oil, cold-pressed
225g (8oz) calf's liver, thinly sliced
1 tablespoon fresh wheatgerm

**Serves 2**
Sauté the onion in the oil until it is soft. Add the liver, sauté for about 1 minute, turn over, add the wheatgerm and sauté for a further minute. Serve with slices of apple and a green salad.

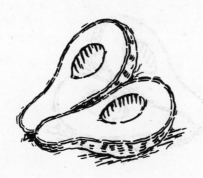

## Day 3

*On Awakening*   1 or 2 glasses of water

*Breakfast*   1 or 2 oranges
5 dried apricots soaked overnight (use sun-dried not sulphur-dried fruit)
Breakfast cereal with 1 tablespoon of wheatgerm
1 glass of health drink of your choice or whole milk. Vitamin and mineral supplements

*Lunch*   1 piece of fresh fruit of your choice (optional)
Date and Avocado Salad
1 glass of whole milk

*Dinner*   1 piece of fresh fruit of your choice
Lemon Chicken Casserole with green, leafy vegetables and jacket potato (optional)
1 glass of whole milk and vitamin and mineral supplements

*Before Bed*   Cod-liver Cocktail (see page 78)

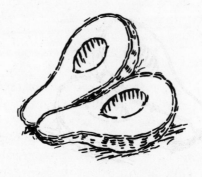

## Date and Avocado Salad

*Serves 1-2*

225g (8oz/1 cup) cottage cheese
½ lettuce, shredded
½ avocado pear, stoned, peeled and
  diced
6 dates, stoned
1 tablespoon peanut butter

Place the cottage cheese on a bed of lettuce and arrange the diced avocado around it. Fill each stoned date with peanut butter and position them on top of the cottage cheese.

## Lemon Chicken Casserole

*Serves 2*

2 chicken pieces (legs or thighs)
1 tablespoon flour
15g (½oz) mock butter (see page 75)
1 teaspoon chopped onion
2 lean rashers bacon, chopped
6 tablespoons chicken stock
grated rind and juice of 1 lemon
1 bay leaf
freshly ground black pepper to taste

Coat the chicken pieces in the flour. Heat the mock butter in a pan, add the chicken pieces and 'seal' the juices over a moderate heat for about 7 minutes. Remove the chicken. Cook the onion and chopped bacon in the fat for 5 minutes, adding any remaining flour and cook for a further 2 minutes. Pour in the stock and slowly bring to the boil, stirring all the time. Add the lemon rind, juice and bay leaf and finally the chicken. Season to taste with freshly ground black pepper and simmer over a low heat until tender.

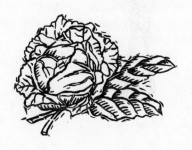

# Day 4

On Awakening  1 or 2 glasses of water

Breakfast  1 or 2 oranges
Poached or scrambled egg on 1 or 2 slices of wholemeal toast or breakfast cereal with 1 tablespoon of wheatgerm
1 glass of health drink of your choice or whole milk. Vitamin and mineral supplements

Lunch  1 piece of fresh fruit of your choice (optional)
Nut Salad
1 glass of whole milk

Dinner  1 piece of fresh fruit of your choice
Ocean Salad
1 glass of whole milk and vitamin and mineral supplements

Before Bed  Cod-liver Cocktail (see page 78)

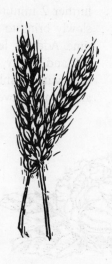

## Nut Salad

*Serves 2*

25g (1oz/1 cup) watercress
25g (1oz/1 cup) lettuce, chopped into
    pieces
100g (4oz/1 cup) celery, chopped
100g (4oz/1 cup) red pepper, diced
2 large tomatoes, sliced
salad dressing of your choice (see
    pages 179–81)
100g (4oz/1 cup) nuts, unsalted and
    ground

Mix all the salad vegetables together and toss in the salad dressing. Sprinkle with the ground nuts and serve.

## Ocean Salad

*Serves 2*

100g (4oz) squid, thinly sliced
225g (8oz) mussels, cooked
50g (2oz) shrimps, peeled
½ onion, finely chopped
2 tomatoes sliced
25g (1oz) watercress
25g (1oz) lettuce, chopped
1 small clove garlic, crushed
2 tablespoons chopped parsley
freshly ground black pepper to taste

Cook the squid in a pan of boiling water for 2 to 3 minutes, remove and drain. Mix together with the other ingredients, toss in the salad dressing of your choice (see pages 179–81) and serve.

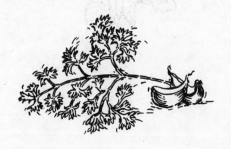

## Day 5

*On Awakening*   1 or 2 glasses of water

*Breakfast*   1 or 2 oranges or 1 small bowl of fresh raspberries or strawberries with whole milk
Breakfast cereal with 1 tablespoon of wheatgerm
1 glass of health drink of your choice or whole milk. Vitamin and mineral supplements

*Lunch*   1 piece of fresh fruit of your choice (optional)
Fruit and Seafood Salad
1 glass of whole milk

*Dinner*   1 piece of fresh fruit of your choice
Savoury Nut Loaf with vegetables of your choice or side salad of your choice
1 glass of whole milk and vitamin and mineral supplements

*Before Bed*   Cod-liver Cocktail (see page 78)

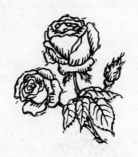

## Fruit and Seafood Salad

½ cantaloupe melon
50g (2oz) grapes, halved and
   deseeded
50g (2oz) prawns or shrimps, peeled
25g (1oz) Edam cheese, cubed

**Serves 1**
Remove the seeds from the melon and
scoop out the flesh, leaving the shell
approximately 1cm (½ in.) thick. Chop
the flesh and combine with the other
ingredients. Pile the mixture into the
melon shell and serve.

## Savoury Nut Loaf

275g (10oz/2 cups) mixed nuts,
   chopped
175g (6oz) wholewheat breadcrumbs
100g (4oz/1 cup) celery, chopped
100g (4oz/¾ cup) onion, finely
   chopped
2 eggs
300ml (10 fl oz/1 cup) fresh tomato
   juice
3 tablespoons vegetable oil, cold-
   pressed
10g (¼oz/¼ cup) fresh parsley,
   chopped
freshly ground black pepper to taste

**Serves 3–4**
Mix all the ingredients together thoroughly.
Pack the mixture evenly into a greased
loaf tin and bake under a low heat until
the loaf is firm and cooked through.
Loosen the sides with a knife and turn
out on to a serving dish. Serve with a
side salad or vegetables of your choice.

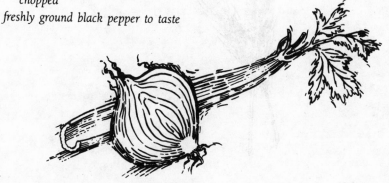

## Day 6

*On Awakening*  1 or 2 glasses of water

*Breakfast*  1 or 2 oranges
Poached or scrambled egg on 1 or 2 slices of wholemeal toast or breakfast cereal with 1 tablespoon of wheatgerm
1 glass of health drink of your choice or whole milk. Vitamin and mineral supplements

*Lunch*  1 piece of fresh fruit of your choice (optional)
Savoury Fruit Salad
1 glass of whole milk

*Dinner*  1 piece of fresh fruit of your choice
Chilli con Carne with brown rice or spinach and broccoli
1 glass of whole milk and vitamin and mineral supplements

*Before Bed*  Cod-liver Cocktail (see page 78)

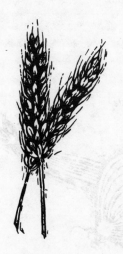

## Savoury Fruit Salad

*Serves 1*

150g (5oz) apples, unpeeled, cored
   and diced
75g (3oz) carrots, grated
salad dressing of your choice (see
   pages 179–81)
40g (1½oz) raisins

Toss the apple and carrot in the salad dressing. Top with the raisins and serve with either tuna, salmon or cottage cheese.

## Chilli con Carne

*Serves 4*

450g (1lb) minced beef
3 medium onions, chopped
1 tablespoon chilli powder
225g (8oz) fresh tomatoes, skinned
600ml (1 pint) meat stock
175g (6oz) cooked (but not drained)
   red kidney beans
1 tablespoon brewers' yeast

Place the minced beef in a large pan over a low heat and stir until the mince is brown. Add the chopped onion and chilli powder and stir well. Add the tomatoes and the stock. Cover with a lid and simmer over a very low heat for between 30 and 45 minutes. Stir in the cooked kidney beans and add just enough cooking water to top up. Add the brewers' yeast and mix thoroughly just before serving. Traditionally, chilli con carne is served with rice, but you may prefer to serve it with spinach and broccoli.

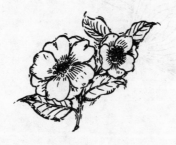

# Day 7

*On Awakening*  1 or 2 glasses of water

*Breakfast*  1 or 2 oranges
Breakfast cereal with 1 tablespoon of wheatgerm
1 glass of health drink of your choice or whole milk. Vitamin and mineral supplements

*Lunch*  1 piece of fresh fruit of your choice (optional)
Salad Supreme
1 glass of whole milk

*Dinner*  1 piece of fresh fruit of your choice
Chicken Livers with Mushrooms with brown rice and side salad of your choice
1 glass of whole milk and vitamin and mineral supplements

*Before Bed*  Cod-liver Cocktail (see page 78)

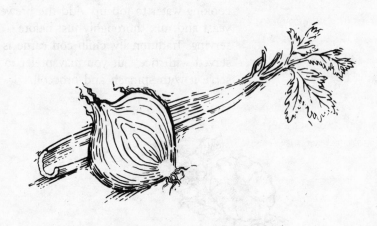

## Salad Supreme

*Serves 1*

2 eggs, hard-boiled and shelled
1 tablespoon plain yogurt
¼ teaspoon French mustard
freshly ground black pepper to taste
25g (1oz) lettuce, shredded
25g (1oz) cucumber, sliced
50g (2oz) red pepper, sliced
1 stick celery, chopped
3 spring onions (scallions),
   chopped
salad dressing of your choice (see
   pages 179–81)

Mash the eggs until smooth. Mix in the yogurt, mustard and freshly ground black pepper to taste. Toss all the remaining ingredients in the salad dressing. Place the egg mixture in the centre of the plate and arrange the salad around it.

## Chicken Livers with Mushrooms

*Serves 2–3*

50g (2oz/¼ cup) mock butter (see
   page 75)
350g (12oz) chicken livers, washed
   and cut into pieces
100g (4oz/2 cups) mushrooms, sliced
2 tablespoons finely chopped onion
pinch of paprika
freshly ground black pepper to taste

Melt the mock butter in a pan and sauté the chicken livers, mushrooms and onion over a very low heat for about 5 minutes or until cooked. Add the paprika and black pepper to taste. Serve on a bed of brown rice with a side salad of your choice. A green salad is good with this meal.

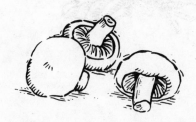

# Day 8

| | |
|---|---|
| *On Awakening* | 1 or 2 glasses of water |
| *Breakfast* | 1 or 2 oranges<br>Breakfast cereal with 1 tablespoon of wheatgerm<br>1 glass of health drink of your choice or whole milk. Vitamin and mineral supplements |
| *Lunch* | 1 piece of fresh fruit of your choice (optional)<br>Cottage Cheese Salad<br>1 glass of whole milk |
| *Dinner* | 1 piece of fresh fruit of your choice<br>Halibut with Sesame Seeds with vegetables of your choice and side salad of your choice<br>1 glass of whole milk and vitamin and mineral supplements |
| *Before Bed* | Cod-liver Cocktail (see page 78) |

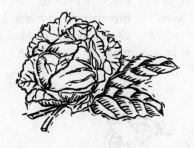

## Cottage Cheese Salad

*Serves 1–2*

50g (2oz/½ cup) celery, chopped
100g (4oz/¼ cup) radishes, diced
25g (1oz/¼ cup) red pepper, diced
2 teaspoons grated onion
salad dressing of your choice (see
    pages 179–81)
100g (4oz/½ cup) cottage cheese

Toss all the salad ingredients in the salad dressing. Serve with the cottage cheese.

## Halibut with Sesame Seeds

*Serves 2*

2 halibut cutlets
2 teaspoons vegetable oil, cold-pressed
freshly ground black pepper to taste
65g (2½oz) wholewheat breadcrumbs
2 tablespoons sesame seeds
¼ teaspoon thyme
2 tablespoons mock butter (see page
    75), melted

Arrange the cutlets on a foil-covered grill pan. Sprinkle with black pepper and pour over the vegetable oil. Mix together the breadcrumbs, sesame seeds, thyme and mock butter and spread evenly on top of the cutlets. Grill under a low heat until fish flakes easily. Serve with vegetables and side salad of your choice.

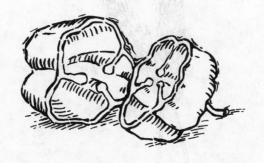

# Day 9

*On Awakening*  1 or 2 glasses of water

*Breakfast*  1 or 2 oranges or 1 small bowl of fresh raspberries or strawberries
with whole milk
Poached or scrambled egg on 1 or 2 slices of wholemeal toast or
breakfast cereal with 1 tablespoon of wheatgerm
1 glass of health drink of your choice or whole milk. Vitamin and
mineral supplements

*Lunch*  1 piece of fresh fruit of your choice (optional)
Seafood Salad with Rice
1 glass of whole milk

*Dinner*  1 piece of fresh fruit of your choice
Honeyed Chicken with Orange and side salad of your choice
1 glass of whole milk and vitamin and mineral supplements

*Before Bed*  Cod-liver Cocktail (see page 78)

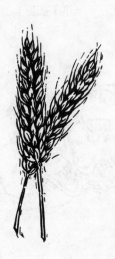

## Seafood Salad with Rice

Serves 1–2

120g (4½oz) cooked brown rice
50g (2oz) prawns, peeled
25g (1oz) mushrooms, finely sliced
salad dressing of your choice
  (see pages 179–81)
watercress to garnish (optional)

Mix the rice, prawns and mushrooms and toss in the salad dressing. Garnish with sprigs of watercress and serve.

## Honeyed Chicken with Orange

Serves 1–2

A knob of mock butter (see page 75)
2 chicken pieces
juice of 1 large orange
2 teaspoons honey

Spread the mock butter on the chicken pieces, sprinkle with black pepper and grill under a moderate heat for 30 minutes or until cooked. When ready, pour away the excess oil.
Mix the orange juice and honey together and pour over the chicken. Return to the grill, under a low heat for a further 5 minutes. Serve with a salad.

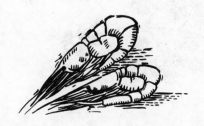

## Day 10

| | |
|---|---|
| *On Awakening* | 1 or 2 glasses of water |
| *Breakfast* | 1 or 2 oranges<br>5 dried apricots soaked overnight<br>Breakfast cereal with 1 tablespoon of wheatgerm<br>1 glass of health drink of your choice or whole milk. Vitamin and mineral supplements |
| *Lunch* | 1 piece of fresh fruit of your choice (optional)<br>Pilchard Salad<br>1 glass of whole milk |
| *Dinner* | 1 piece of fresh fruit of your choice<br>Anita's Risotto<br>1 glass of whole milk and vitamin and mineral supplements |
| *Before Bed* | Cod-liver Cocktail (see page 78) |

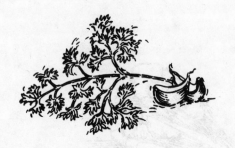

## Pilchard Salad

100g (4oz) pilchards or sardines,
    cooked or tinned
100g (4oz) lettuce, shredded
50g (2oz) white cabbage, shredded
50g (2oz) red pepper, chopped
2 radishes, sliced
½ red apple, cored and chopped
½ orange, peeled and segmented
50g (2oz) melon, chopped
salad dressing of your choice (see
    pages 179–81)

*Serves 1*

Toss all the ingredients, except the
pilchards, in the salad dressing. Add the
pilchards and serve.

## Anita's Risotto

225g (8oz/1 cup) uncooked brown
    rice
1 onion, chopped
1 clove garlic, minced
600ml (1 pint) vegetable stock or
    water
pinch of saffron
½ teaspoon rosemary
3 tablespoons fresh, finely chopped
    parsley
50g (2oz/½ cup) cheddar cheese,
    grated
50g (2oz/½ cup) mixed sunflower
    and pumpkin seeds
freshly ground black pepper to taste

*Serves 2–3*

Sauté the onion, garlic and rice in a little
vegetable oil (cold-pressed) until soft. Add
the stock or water, saffron, herbs and
freshly ground black pepper to taste. Cook
slowly over a low heat, adding a little
more stock or water if necessary. When
the rice is tender and all the liquid has
been absorbed, stir in the seeds, sprinkle
with cheese and serve.

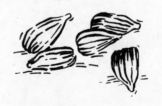

# Day 11

| | |
|---|---|
| *On Awakening* | 1 or 2 glasses of water |
| *Breakfast* | 1 or 2 oranges<br>Breakfast cereal with 1 tablespoon of wheatgerm<br>1 glass of health drink of your choice or whole milk. Vitamin and mineral supplements |
| *Lunch* | 1 piece of fresh fruit of your choice (optional)<br>Broad Bean Salad (see page 107)<br>1 glass of whole milk |
| *Dinner* | 1 piece of fresh fruit of your choice<br>Lamb with Lemon and Ginger with jacket potato and green, leafy vegetables of your choice<br>1 glass of whole milk and vitamin and mineral supplements |
| *Before Bed* | Cod-liver Cocktail (see page 78) |

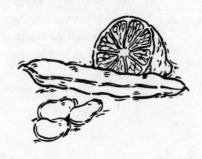

# Lamb with Lemon and Ginger

*Serves 2*

2–4 lamb chops or slices from leg or
   shoulder of lamb
4 tablespoons vegetable oil, cold-
   pressed
2 tablespoons lemon juice
1 teaspoon ground ginger
freshly ground black pepper to taste

Mix the oil, lemon juice, ginger and
pepper together. Place the chops or pieces
of lamb in a shallow dish and pour the
marinade over them. Leave to marinate for
approximately 3 hours, turning
occasionally.

Place the chops or pieces of lamb on a
grill pan, and pour the marinade over
them. Grill over a low heat, basting with
the marinade regularly, until cooked.

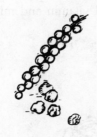

## Day 12

*On Awakening*   1 or 2 glasses water

*Breakfast*   1 or 2 oranges
Poached or scrambled egg on 1 or 2 slices of wholemeal toast or
breakfast cereal with 1 tablespoon of wheatgerm
1 glass of health drink of your choice or whole milk. Vitamin and
mineral supplements

*Lunch*   1 piece of fresh fruit of your choice (optional)
Tuna and Red Kidney Bean Salad (see page 109)
1 glass of whole milk

*Dinner*   1 piece of fresh fruit of your choice
Venetian Fish Pie with side salad of your choice
1 glass of whole milk and vitamin and mineral supplements

*Before Bed*   Cod-liver Cocktail (see page 78)

## Venetian Fish Pie

freshly ground black pepper to taste
1 bunch fresh broccoli
2 cod or haddock cutlets or fillets,
   poached
¼ pint cheese sauce
1 tablespoon fresh wholemeal
   breadcrumbs
1 tablespoon grated cheese
knob mock butter (see page 75)

To make the Cheese Sauce
1 tablespoon butter
1 tablespoon flour
150ml (5 fl oz) milk
3 tablespoons grated cheese
pinch mustard powder

Serves 2
Steam the broccoli, drain thoroughly and place it in a buttered, shallow, ovenproof dish. Season with freshly ground black pepper. Melt the butter in a pan, stir in the flour, thoroughly, then gradually add the milk and bring to the boil, stirring all the time. Cook for 3 minutes, remove from the heat and stir in the cheese and mustard powder. Continue to stir until the cheese has melted. Place the poached fish on the broccoli. Pour the cheese sauce over. Mix the breadcrumbs and cheese together and sprinkle on top. Dot with the mock butter, grill under a low heat for a few minutes until the cheese topping has melted.

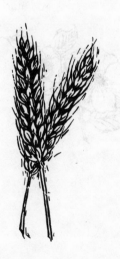

# Day 13

On Awakening    1 or 2 glasses of water

Breakfast    1 or 2 oranges
Breakfast cereal with 1 tablespoon of wheatgerm
1 glass of health drink of your choice or whole milk. Vitamin and mineral supplements

Lunch    1 piece of fresh fruit of your choice (optional)
Date and Avocado Salad (see page 111)
1 glass of whole milk

Dinner    1 piece of fresh fruit of your choice
Calf's Liver à L'Orange with brown rice and side salad of your choice
1 glass of whole milk and vitamin and mineral supplements

Before Bed    Cod-liver Cocktail (see page 78)

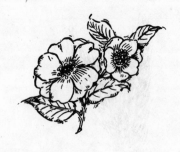

## Calf's Liver à L'Orange

*Serves 2*

½ large onion
1 clove garlic
pinch cayenne pepper
pinch mustard powder
freshly ground black pepper
4 slices calf's liver
1 tablespoon wholemeal flour
1 tablespoon sunflower oil
150ml (5 fl oz/½ cup) stock or water
a little red wine, to taste
pinch of parsley
pinch of thyme
½ large orange, sliced

Chop the onion and crush the garlic and put them to one side. Add the pinch of cayenne pepper, mustard and black pepper to the flour. Coat the liver slices with the seasoned flour and fry in the oil for 1 or 2 minutes or until they are cooked. Remove them from the pan and keep warm.

Next, add the onion and the garlic to the juices and the oil, and cook gently until soft. Add the stock, wine and herbs and simmer for a few minutes. Spoon the mixture over the liver. Serve with brown rice and a green salad and garnish with the orange slices.

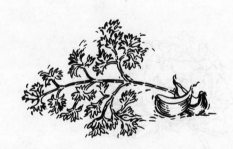

## Day 14

**On Awakening**  1 or 2 glasses of water

**Breakfast**  1 or 2 oranges
Poached or scrambled egg on 1 or 2 slices of wholemeal toast or breakfast cereal with 1 tablespoon of wheatgerm
1 glass of health drink of your choice or whole milk. Vitamin and mineral supplements

**Lunch**  1 piece of fresh fruit of your choice (optional)
Nut Salad (see page 113)
1 glass of whole milk

**Dinner**  1 piece of fresh fruit of your choice
Grilled Chicken with Lemon and jacket potato (optional) and green, leafy vegetables
1 glass of whole milk and vitamin and mineral supplements

**Before Bed**  Cod-liver Cocktail (see page 78)

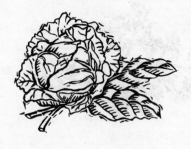

132

## Grilled Chicken with Lemon

**Serves 1–2**

juice of 1 lemon freshly squeezed
2 chicken pieces (thighs)
vegetable oil
freshly ground black pepper to taste

Sprinkle the lemon juice over the chicken pieces, brush with oil, and season with freshly ground black pepper. Place the chicken thighs skin side downwards in a pan and grill under a low to medium heat for about 10 minutes. Turn the chicken over, brush with more oil and continue grilling for about 20 minutes, basting with the juices, until cooked. Squeeze over any remaining lemon juice and serve.

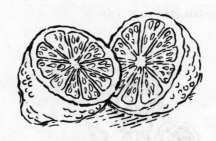

## Day 15

*On Awakening*   1 or 2 glasses water

*Breakfast*   1 or 2 oranges
5 dried apricots soaked overnight
Breakfast cereal with 1 tablespoon of wheatgerm
1 glass of health drink of your choice or whole milk. Vitamin and mineral supplements

*Lunch*   1 piece of fresh fruit of your choice (optional)
Fruit and Seafood Salad (see page 115)
1 glass of whole milk

*Dinner*   1 piece of fresh fruit of your choice
Carrot Loaf with vegetables of your choice or side salad of your choice
1 glass of whole milk and vitamin and mineral supplements

*Before Bed*   Cod-liver Cocktail (see page 78)

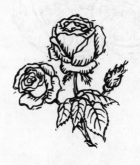

# Carrot Loaf

150g (5oz/¾ cup) carrot, grated
50g (2oz/½ cup) mixed nuts,
  chopped
1 small onion, finely chopped
1 stick celery, chopped
2 tablespoons wholewheat
  breadcrumbs
2 tablespoons chopped fresh parsley
2 tablespoons fresh cream
1 egg, beaten
freshly ground black pepper to taste
2 tablespoons vegetable oil, cold-
  pressed
wholewheat breadcrumbs
2 teaspoons mock butter (see page
  75)

*Serves 2–3*

Combine all the ingredients except the vegetable oil, the second quantity of breadcrumbs and the mock butter. Coat the inside of the loaf tin with vegetable oil and sprinkle the oiled surfaces with the remaining breadcrumbs. Pack the carrot mixture evenly into the loaf tin, dot the top with the mock butter, cover and bake under a low heat for about 45 minutes to 1 hour. Uncover for the last 5 minutes of cooking. Loosen the sides with a knife and turn out on to a serving dish. Serve with a side salad or vegetables of your choice.

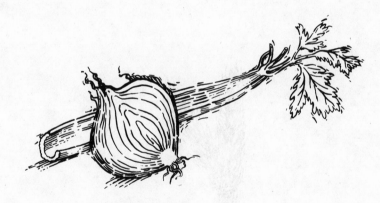

## Day 16

On Awakening   1 or 2 glasses of water

Breakfast   1 or 2 oranges
Breakfast cereal with 1 tablespoon of wheatgerm
1 glass of health drink of your choice or whole milk. Vitamin and mineral supplements

Lunch   1 piece of fresh fruit of your choice (optional)
Savoury Fruit Salad (see page 117)
1 glass of whole milk

Dinner   1 piece of fresh fruit of your choice
Grilled Lemon Sole with jacket potato (optional) and green, leafy vegetables of your choice
1 glass of whole milk and vitamin and mineral supplements

Before Bed   Cod-liver Cocktail (see page 78)

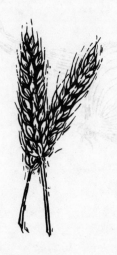

136

## Grilled Lemon Sole

25g (1oz) mock butter (see page 75)
2 medium-sized lemon soles
1 tablespoon freshly squeezed lemon
   juice
freshly ground black pepper to taste

Serves 2

Spread the butter over a piece of foil large enough to enclose the fish completely. Place the fish in the centre, sprinkle with the lemon juice and season with freshly ground black pepper. Fold the foil into an envelope and seal. Grill under a low heat until cooked. Serve with spinach or Brussels sprouts (lightly steamed) or any vegetable of your choice.

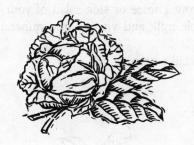

# Day 17

*On Awakening*  1 or 2 glasses of water

*Breakfast*  1 or 2 oranges or 1 small bowl of fresh raspberries or strawberries with whole milk
Poached or scrambled egg on 1 or 2 slices of wholemeal toast or breakfast cereal with 1 tablespoon of wheatgerm
1 glass of health drink of your choice or whole milk. Vitamin and mineral supplements

*Lunch*  1 piece of fresh fruit of your choice (optional)
Salad Supreme (see page 119)
1 glass of whole milk

*Dinner*  1 piece of fresh fruit of your choice
Beef Vegetable Burgers with jacket potato and green, leafy vegetables of your choice or side salad of your choice
1 glass of whole milk and vitamin and mineral supplements

*Before Bed*  Cod-liver Cocktail (see page 78)

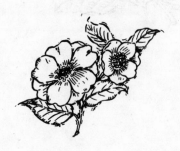

## Beef Vegetable Burgers

*Serves 4*

225g (8oz) minced beef
175g (6oz/1 cup) carrots, grated
175g (6oz/1 cup) potatoes, unpeeled
  and grated
50g (2oz/½ cup) celery, finely
  chopped
2 tablespoons finely chopped onion
2 tablespoons fresh chopped parsley
1 egg beaten
65ml (2½ fl oz/¼ cup) milk
25g (1oz) wheatgerm
freshly ground black pepper to taste

Mix all the ingredients together. Divide the mixture into 8 equal portions and shape them into burgers. Place them on a buttered baking tray. Bake in a low to moderate oven until cooked, but before they brown. Serve with jacket potatoes and either steamed, green vegetables or a side salad of your choice.

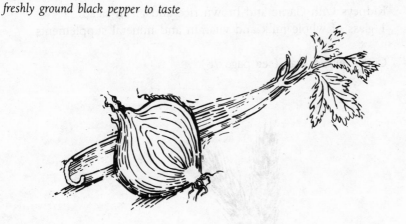

## Day 18

On Awakening    1 or 2 glasses of water

Breakfast    1 or 2 oranges
Breakfast cereal with 1 tablespoon of wheatgerm
1 glass of health drink of your choice or whole milk. Vitamin and mineral supplements

Lunch    1 piece of fresh fruit of your choice (optional)
Cottage Cheese Salad (see page 121)
1 glass of whole milk

Dinner    1 piece of fresh fruit of your choice
Kidneys with Garlic and brown rice and green salad
1 glass of whole milk and vitamin and mineral supplements

Before Bed    Cod-liver Cocktail (see page 78)

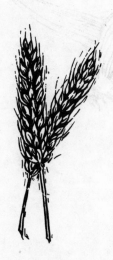

## Kidneys with Garlic

*Serves 2*

4 lambs' kidneys
2 large cloves garlic
freshly ground black pepper to taste
½ tablespoon sunflower oil, cold-
    pressed
juice of half a lemon

Skin and core the kidneys before cutting into 1-cm (½-inch) pieces. Chop the garlic, add to the kidneys, season with freshly ground black pepper and fry in oil over low-to-medium heat for 4 to 5 minutes. Add the lemon juice and serve on a bed of lightly steamed spinach or any green, leafy vegetables.

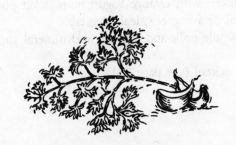

## Day 19

| | |
|---|---|
| *On Awakening* | 1 or 2 glasses of water |
| *Breakfast* | 1 or 2 oranges<br>Poached or scrambled egg on 1 or 2 slices of wholemeal toast or breakfast cereal with 1 tablespoon of wheatgerm<br>1 glass of health drink of your choice or whole milk. Vitamin and mineral supplements |
| *Lunch* | 1 piece of fresh fruit of your choice (optional)<br>Seafood Salad with Rice (see page 123)<br>1 glass of whole milk |
| *Dinner* | 1 piece of fresh fruit of your choice<br>Grilled Chicken with Orange Yogurt with jacket potato (optional) and broccoli or any green, leafy vegetable<br>1 glass of whole milk and vitamin and mineral supplements |
| *Before Bed* | Cod-liver Cocktail (see page 78) |

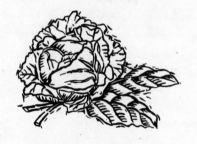

## Grilled Chicken with Orange Yogurt

1 medium onion, finely chopped
juice of 1 medium orange, and half
   the rind
4 fl oz chicken stock or water
sprig of thyme (preferably fresh)
2 chicken thighs
freshly ground black pepper to taste
vegetable oil
½ teaspoon cornflour
1 tablespoon plain yogurt

*Serves 2*
Place the onion, orange rind and juice,
stock or water and thyme in a small pan.
Slowly bring to the boil, cover and
simmer for 30 minutes.

Meanwhile, season the chicken thighs
with freshly ground black pepper and
brush with a little oil. Grill, turning
occasionally until cooked.

Combine the cornflour with a little cold
water and stir this into the orange juice
mixture. Slowly bring to the boil and
simmer for 2 minutes, stirring all the time.
Remove from the heat and continue to
stir. When the mixture has cooled and is
pleasantly warm, stir in the yogurt. Serve
the grilled chicken portions on warm
plates and pour over the orange yogurt
sauce. Serve with steamed broccoli.

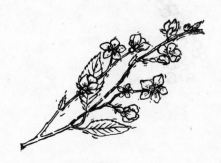

# Day 20

On Awakening   1 or 2 glasses of water

Breakfast   1 or 2 oranges
Breakfast cereal with 1 tablespoon of wheatgerm
1 glass of health drink of your choice or whole milk. Vitamin and mineral supplements

Lunch   1 piece of fresh fruit of your choice (optional)
Pilchard Salad (see page 125)
1 glass of whole milk

Dinner   1 piece of fresh fruit of your choice
Potato and Egg Bake with salad of your choice
1 glass of whole milk and vitamin and mineral supplements

Before Bed   Cod-liver Cocktail (see page 78)

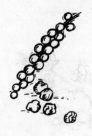

## Potato and Egg Bake

2 large baking potatoes, washed
2 eggs, separated
25g (1oz) cheese, grated
freshly ground black pepper to taste

*Serves 2*

Prick the potatoes with a skewer and bake in a low to moderate oven until the centres are soft.

Cut each potato in half and scoop out the flesh into a bowl. Keep the four shells. Mash the flesh thoroughly, stir in the beaten egg yolks and sprinkle with pepper. Beat the egg whites until stiff and gently fold in to the potato mixture with a spoon. Scoop the mixture into the potato shells, sprinkle with grated cheese and bake until they are about to brown. Serve with a salad of your choice.

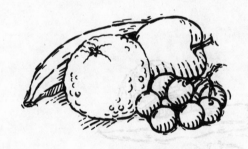

# Day 21

*On Awakening*   1 or 2 glasses of water

*Breakfast*   1 or 2 oranges
Breakfast cereal with 1 tablespoon of wheatgerm
1 glass of health drink of your choice or whole milk. Vitamin and mineral supplements

*Lunch*   1 piece of fresh fruit of your choice (optional)
Broad Bean Salad (see page 107)
1 glass of whole milk

*Dinner*   1 piece of fresh fruit of your choice
Baked Trout with Oatmeal and jacket potato (optional) and fresh peas or side salad of your choice
1 glass of whole milk and vitamin and mineral supplements

*Before Bed*   Cod-liver Cocktail (see page 78)

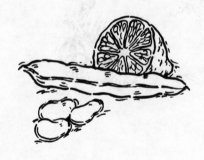

## Baked Trout with Oatmeal

20g (¾oz) oatmeal
25g (1oz) almonds, chopped
freshly ground black pepper to taste
2 fresh trout, cleaned
25g (1oz) mock butter (see page 75),
   melted

*Serves 2*

Mix the oatmeal with the chopped almonds and sprinkle with pepper. Brush one side of each trout with the melted butter, then press the buttered side of the fish on to the oatmeal and nut mixture, then lay the fish on a greased oven dish, oatmeal-side downwards. Brush the top of the fish with melted butter. Sprinkle over the remaining oatmeal and nut mixture, pressing it so that it adheres to the surface of the fish. Pour over the remaining butter. Bake in a low-to-moderate oven until cooked. Serve with either peas and jacket potatoes or a side salad.

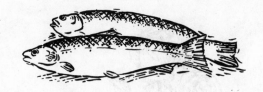

## Day 22

<table>
<tr><td>On Awakening</td><td>1 or 2 glasses of water</td></tr>
<tr><td>Breakfast</td><td>1 or 2 oranges<br>Poached or scrambled egg on 1 or 2 slices of wholemeal toast or breakfast cereal with 1 tablespoon of wheatgerm<br>1 glass of health drink of your choice or whole milk. Vitamin and mineral supplements</td></tr>
<tr><td>Lunch</td><td>1 piece of fresh fruit of your choice (optional)<br>Tuna and Red Kidney Bean Salad (see page 109)<br>1 glass of whole milk</td></tr>
<tr><td>Dinner</td><td>1 piece of fresh fruit of your choice<br>Meat Loaf with green, leafy vegetables of your choice or side salad of your choice<br>1 glass of whole milk and vitamin and mineral supplements</td></tr>
<tr><td>Before Bed</td><td>Cod-liver Cocktail (see page 78)</td></tr>
</table>

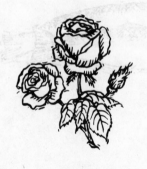

## Meat Loaf

### Serves 4–6

450g (1lb) minced beef

175g (6oz) fresh wholewheat breadcrumbs

225g (8oz) carrots, grated

1 small onion, diced

½ red pepper, cored and finely chopped

1 tablespoon Worcestershire sauce

1 tablespoon fresh tomato juice

1 teaspoon French mustard

1 teaspoon mixed herbs

1 large egg, beaten

freshly ground black pepper to taste

Combine all the ingredients and spread the mixture evenly in a loaf or cake tin lined with greaseproof paper, levelling the top with a fork. Cover with foil. Bake in a low to medium oven until cooked. Serve either hot with green, leafy vegetables or cold with a side salad.

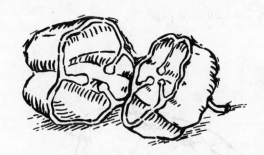

# Day 23

*On Awakening*  1 or 2 glasses of water

*Breakfast*  1 or 2 oranges
5 dried apricots soaked overnight
Breakfast cereal with 1 tablespoon wheatgerm
1 glass of health drink of your choice or whole milk. Vitamin and mineral supplements

*Lunch*  1 piece of fresh fruit of your choice (optional)
Date and Avocado Salad (see page 111)
1 glass of whole milk

*Dinner*  1 piece of fresh fruit of your choice
Curried Liver and Kidneys with jacket potato (optional) and green, leafy vegetables of your choice or side salad of your choice
1 glass of whole milk and vitamin and mineral supplements

*Before Bed*  Cod-liver Cocktail (see page 78)

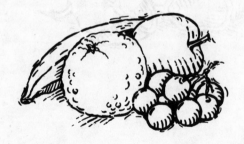

# Curried Liver and Kidneys

Serves 2

3–4 lambs' kidneys
2 teaspoons vegetable oil, cold-pressed
½ teaspoon curry powder
½ teaspoon French mustard
pinch sea salt (optional)
225g (8oz) calf's liver, thinly sliced
1 tablespoon wholewheat flour
6 tablespoons stock or water

Skin, core and slice the kidneys. Add the oil to a pan, stir in the curry powder, mustard, and salt (if necessary) and fry gently for 5 minutes. Add the liver and kidneys and sauté for 2 minutes. Stir in the flour, add the stock or water, cover and simmer over a low heat for 10 minutes.

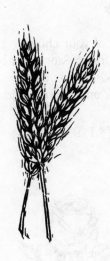

## Day 24

On Awakening   1 or 2 glasses of water

Breakfast   1 or 2 oranges or 1 small bowl of fresh raspberries or strawberries
with whole milk
Breakfast cereal with 1 tablespoon of wheatgerm
1 glass of health drink of your choice or whole milk. Vitamin and
mineral supplements

Lunch   1 piece of fresh fruit of your choice (optional)
Nut Salad (see page 113)
1 glass of whole milk

Dinner   1 piece of fresh fruit of your choice
Fillets of Fish with Orange Sauce and broccoli or any green, leafy
vegetable or side salad of your choice .
1 glass of whole milk and vitamin and mineral supplements

Before Bed   Cod-liver Cocktail (see page 78)

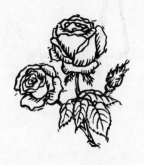

## Fillets of Fish with Orange Sauce

**Serves 2**

450g (1lb) fish fillets of your choice
2 tablespoons vegetable oil, cold-
   pressed
200ml (7 fl oz) plain yogurt
6 tablespoons freshly squeezed
   orange juice

Arrange the fillets on a foil-covered grill pan. Cover with the oil and grill slowly under a low heat until cooked. Prepare the orange sauce by blending together the yogurt and the orange juice until smooth. Pour over the cooked fillets and serve with steamed broccoli and side salad of your choice.

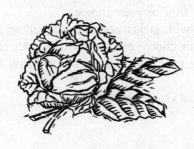

# Day 25

*On Awakening*   1 or 2 glasses of water

*Breakfast*   1 or 2 oranges
Poached or scrambled egg on 1 or 2 slices of wholemeal toast or breakfast cereal with 1 tablespoon of wheatgerm
1 glass of health drink of your choice or whole milk. Vitamin and mineral supplements

*Lunch*   1 piece of fresh fruit of your choice (optional)
Fruit and Seafood Salad (see page 115)
1 glass of whole milk

*Dinner*   1 piece of fresh fruit of your choice
Chicken Peking with jacket potato (optional) and green, leafy vegetables of your choice or side salad of your choice
1 glass of whole milk and vitamin and mineral supplements

*Before Bed*   Cod-liver Cocktail (see page 78)

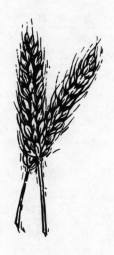

## Chicken Peking

*2 chicken pieces (thighs are ideal)*
*2 tablespoons honey*
*25g (1oz) mock butter (see page 75)*
*1 teaspoon soy sauce*

*Serves 1–2*

Mix the honey, mock butter and soy sauce together and coat the chicken with the mixture. Put the chicken in an oven-proof dish lined with cooking foil, and bake in a pre-heated oven at 450 deg F/Gas Mark 8 for 45 minutes, although a low heat is preferred.

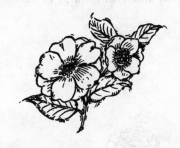

## Day 26

*On Awakening*    1 or 2 glasses water

*Breakfast*    1 or 2 oranges
Breakfast cereal of your choice with 1 tablespoon of wheatgerm
1 glass of health drink of your choice or whole milk. Vitamin and
mineral supplements

*Lunch*    1 piece of fresh fruit of your choice (optional)
Savoury Fruit Salad (see page 117)
1 glass of whole milk

*Dinner*    1 piece of fresh fruit of your choice
Rice with Eggs and Prawns and side salad of your choice
1 glass of whole milk and vitamin and minerals supplements

*Before Bed*    Cod-liver Cocktail (see page 78)

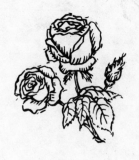

## Rice with Eggs and Prawns

*Serves 2–3*

175g (6oz) uncooked brown rice
1 onion, finely sliced
1 tablespoon vegetable oil, cold-
  pressed
100g (4oz) beansprouts
2.5cm (1in) length fresh ginger,
  grated (optional)
100g (4oz) fresh peas or sweetcorn
225g (8oz) prawns, shelled
2 tablespoons soy sauce
2 eggs
4 spring onions (scallions),
  chopped

Boil the rice until it is just cooked. Meanwhile, sauté the onion in half the oil until soft, drain and keep hot. Add the beansprouts and the ginger to the remaining oil, which should be warm but not sizzling hot, and, when hot, put these with the onion. Steam the peas or sweetcorn until they are almost cooked but not soft and put them with the other vegetables. Heat the prawns in a little oil, add the soy sauce and keep hot. Beat each egg separately, and pour into an omelette pan with a dash of oil and cook. When you have two omelettes, cut them into ribbons. Arrange the onions, beansprouts, ginger, peas or sweetcorn and prawns on a bed of rice. Top with the omelette ribbons and spring onions. Serve with a side salad of your choice.

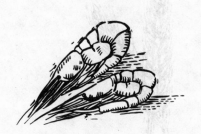

## Day 27

| | |
|---|---|
| *On Awakening* | 1 or 2 glasses water |
| *Breakfast* | 1 or 2 oranges<br>Breakfast cereal with 1 tablespoon of wheatgerm<br>1 glass of health drink of your choice or whole milk. Vitamin and mineral supplements |
| *Lunch* | 1 piece of fresh fruit of your choice (optional)<br>Salad Supreme (see page 119)<br>1 glass of whole milk |
| *Dinner* | 1 piece of fresh fruit of your choice<br>Calf's Liver Loaf with jacket potato (optional) and green, leafy vegetables of your choice<br>1 glass of whole milk and vitamin and mineral supplements |
| *Before Bed* | Cod-liver Cocktail (see page 78) |

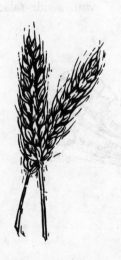

## Calf's Liver Loaf

### Serves 6–8

3 tablespoons vegetable oil, cold-
pressed

450g (1lb) calf's livers, cut into 1-cm
(½-in) slices

50g (2oz/½ cup) onion, finely sliced

25g (1oz/¼ cup) celery, finely sliced

50g (2oz/½ cup) red pepper, finely
sliced

450g (1lb) mince beef

200g (7oz/½ cup) carrot, finely
chopped

1 tablespoon chopped celery leaves

2 tablespoons fresh chopped parsley

2 tablespoons fresh wheatgerm

¼ teaspoon paprika

2 eggs, beaten

Heat the vegetable oil in a pan and sauté the liver for 2 minutes. Remove the liver from the pan, mince finely in a food processor and put to one side. Add more oil to the pan (if necessary), add the onion and, when almost cooked, add the celery and the red pepper and sauté until just tender.

Combine all the ingredients and mix thoroughly. Place in a well-oiled dish, cover and bake in a moderate oven for about 30 minutes. Remove the cover and bake for a further 7 to 8 minutes.

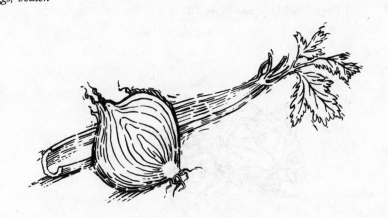

## Day 28

| | |
|---|---|
| *On Awakening* | 1 or 2 glasses of water |
| *Breakfast* | 1 or 2 oranges<br>Poached or scrambled egg with 1 or 2 slices of wholemeal toast or breakfast cereal with 1 tablespoon of wheatgerm<br>1 glass of health drink of your choice or whole milk. Vitamin and mineral supplements |
| *Lunch* | 1 piece of fresh fruit of your choice (optional)<br>Cottage Cheese Salad (see page 121)<br>1 glass of whole milk |
| *Dinner* | 1 piece of fresh fruit of your choice<br>Fish Loaf with green, leafy vegetables of your choice or side salad of your choice<br>1 glass of whole milk and vitamin and mineral supplements |
| *Before Bed* | Cod-liver Cocktail (see page 78) |

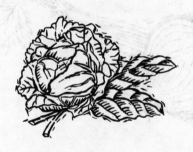

## Fish Loaf

75g (3oz) wholemeal breadcrumbs
150ml (5 fl oz) milk
225g (8oz) fresh (cooked) or tinned
    tuna or salmon, drained
2 eggs, beaten
freshly ground black pepper to taste
1 tablespoon freshly squeezed lemon
    juice
fresh parsley, to garnish
1 tomato, sliced

*Serves 3–4*
Blend all the ingredients together, except
the parsley and the tomato. Pack the
mixture into a well-oiled loaf tin. Bake
under a low heat until set and fairly firm.
Garnish with the parsley and tomato
slices and serve either hot or cold.

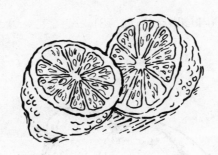

## Day 29

| | |
|---|---|
| *On Awakening* | 1 or 2 glasses of water |
| *Breakfast* | 1 or 2 oranges<br>5 dried apricots soaked overnight<br>Breakfast cereal with 1 tablespoon of wheatgerm<br>1 glass of health drink of your choice or whole milk. Vitamin and mineral supplements |
| *Lunch* | 1 piece of fresh fruit of your choice (optional)<br>Seafood Salad with rice (see page 123)<br>1 glass of whole milk |
| *Dinner* | 1 piece of fresh fruit of your choice<br>Garlic Chicken with jacket potato (optional) and green, leafy vegetables of your choice or side salad of your choice<br>1 glass of whole milk and vitamin and mineral supplements |
| *Before Bed* | Cod-liver Cocktail (see page 78) |

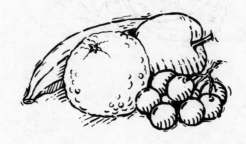

# Garlic Chicken

### Serves 1–2

50g (2oz) mock butter (see page 75)
1 tablespoon freshly squeezed lemon
    juice
1 tablespoon honey
1 clove garlic, crushed
¼ teaspoon mustard powder
¼ teaspoon marjoram
2 chicken pieces

Melt the mock butter in a small pan over a low heat. Stir in the lemon juice, honey, garlic, mustard powder and marjoram. Place the chicken pieces fleshy side upwards on a grill pan lined with foil. Spoon over the mock butter and honey mixture, and leave to marinate for 45 minutes.

Grill the chicken pieces under a moderate heat for 10 to 15 minutes, and then turn over and cook slowly, basting with the juices until cooked. Pierce the thickest part of the flesh and, when the juices run clear, the chicken is cooked.

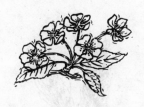

## Day 30

| On Awakening | 1 or 2 glasses of water |
|---|---|

**Breakfast** 1 or 2 oranges or small bowl of fresh raspberries or strawberries with whole milk
Breakfast cereal with 1 tablespoon of wheatgerm
1 glass of health drink of your choice or whole milk. Vitamin and mineral supplements

**Lunch** 1 piece of fresh fruit of your choice (optional)
Pilchard Salad (see page 125)
1 glass of whole milk

**Dinner** 1 piece of fresh fruit of your choice
Soya Bean Roast with jacket potato (optional) and green, leafy vegetables of your choice or side salad of your choice
1 glass of whole milk and vitamin and mineral supplements

**Before Bed** Cod-liver Cocktail (see page 78)

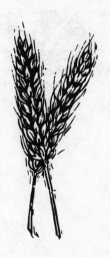

## Soya Bean Roast

*Serves 2–3*

175g (6oz/1 cup) cooked soya beans
175g (6oz/1 cup) carrots, grated
175g (6oz/1 cup) beet, grated
1 onion, grated
1 green pepper, finely chopped
3 tablespoons soya flour
50g (2 oz/½ cup) fresh wheatgerm
85ml (3 fl oz/⅓ cup) fresh tomato
   juice
2 eggs
1 teaspoon parsley
1 teaspoon oregano
½ teaspoon sea salt (optional)

Mix all the ingredients together. Spread the mixture evenly in an oiled loaf tin. Bake at a low heat for 1½ or 2 hours. Serve with a green, leafy vegetable and a jacket potato (optional).

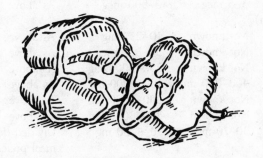

# Supplementation: Nutritional Guidelines

## Vitamins

| Name of Nutrient | Recommended Daily Adult Dose | Anti-Wrinkle Plan Dose | Intake |
|---|---|---|---|
| Vitamin A | 5000 IU | 15 000–25 000 IU | Divided doses with each meal, but not at the same time as iron |
| Vitamin $B_1$ (Thiamine) | 0.9–1.4 mg | 10–500 mg | Divided doses with each meal as part of a B complex formula |
| Vitamin $B_2$ (Riboflavin) | 1.2–1.7 mg | 10–500 mg | As above |
| Vitamin $B_3$ (Niacin) | 13–19 mg | 200–3000 mg | As above |
| Vitamin $B_5$ (Pantothenic acid) | 10–50 mg | 200–3000 mg | As above |
| Vitamin $B_6$ (Pyridoxine) | 1.6–2.5 mg | 10–500 mg | As above |
| Vitamin $B_{12}$ (Cyanocobalamin) | 3–6 mcg | 6–500 mcg | As above |
| Vitamin $B_{15}$ | Not known | 10–250 mg | As above |
| Biotin | Not known | 50–300 mcg | As above |
| Choline | Not known | 250–3000 mg | As above |
| Folic acid | 400–800 mcg | 100–5000 mcg | As above |
| Inositol | Not known | 250–3000 mg | As above |
| PABA | Not known | 200–3000 mg | As above |
| Vitamin C | 30–70 mg | 70–4000 mg | Divided doses with each meal preferably taken with calcium but not at the same time as iron |
| Vitamin D | 400 IU | 400–2500 IU | Divided doses with each meal |
| Vitamin E | 12–15 IU | 400–15 000 IU | Divided doses with each meal, but not at the same time as iron |
| Vitamin K | Not known | 300–500 mcg | Dose to be taken with meal containing some fat or oil |

# Minerals and Trace Elements

| Name of Nutrient | Recommended Daily Adult Dose | Anti-Wrinkle Plan Dose | Intake |
|---|---|---|---|
| Calcium | 800–1200 mg | 1000–2500 mg | Divided doses with each meal as part of a mineral supplement with A and B complex vitamins and/or citric fruits |
| Chromium | Not known | 10–250 mcg | As above |
| Copper | 2 mg | 2 mg | As above |
| Iodine | 100–130 mcg | 3–4 mg | As above |
| Iron | 10–18 mg | 5–10 mg | As above but not at the same time as vitamins A, C and E |
| Magnesium | 300–350 mg | 500–1250 mg (or half the calcium intake) | Divided doses with each meal as part of a mineral supplement |
| Manganese | Not known | 10–50 mg | As above |
| Phosphorus | 800–1000 mg | 2000–5000mg (or no more than twice the amount of calcium) | As above |
| Potassium | Not known | Depends on salt intake; 5000 mg needed daily for each teaspoon of salt consumed | As above |
| Selenium | Not known | 70–400 mcg | As above |
| Sodium | 3–7 g | 1 g or less | |
| Sulphur | Not known | 10–20 mg | Divided doses with each meal as part of a mineral supplement |
| Zinc | 15–20 mg | 15–200 mg | As above |

# Facial Skin Care Programme

*For Dry and Deeply Lined and Wrinkled Skin*

A.M.

- Wash with water only, using 40 splashes of warm, not hot, water followed by 10 cool splashes. Pat dry.
- Apply cider vinegar and water freshener (see page 89) or any non-alcoholic commercial brand, lightly over the face with cotton wool.
- Apply vitamin E oil to face and throat and gently massage in with a water-in-oil cream or fresh, double dairy cream. Leave for 20 minutes before tissuing off.
- Apply unrefined vegetable oil under the eyes and pat in (don't rub).
- Apply make-up.

P.M.

- Remove make-up with unrefined vegetable oil or a suitable water-in-oil cleanser. Apply and wait for one minute before removing with a wet and warm, but not hot, face flannel. Repeat several times until all traces of make-up have gone.
- Apply milk or a suitable oil-in-water emulsion and remove with moistened cotton wool. Repeat.
- Wash with a little soap (see page 87). Rinse thoroughly 15 times in warm water and finish with a cool water splash.
- Apply the Three in One Skin Care Treatment (see page 99). Rinse thoroughly and pat dry.
- Apply petroleum jelly to face and neck and tissue off.
- Apply unrefined vegetable oil under the eyes and pat in.

## Additional Treatments

- Exfoliate with oatmeal once every ten days (see page 99).
- Practise facial exercises a minimum of three times a week (see page 82).
- Apply Anti-Wrinkle and Antioxidant Skin Food (see page 97) to face and neck at least four times a week in addition to normal moisturizing (see page 89).

## *For Dry to Normal/Combination, Slightly Wrinkled Skin*

A.M.

- Wash with the minimum of soap (see page 87). Rinse at least 15 times in warm water, followed by 10 cool water splashes. Pat dry.
- Apply cider vinegar and water freshener (see page 89) or any non-alcoholic commercial freshener, lightly over the face with cotton wool.
- Apply vitamin E oil or any unrefined vegetable oil to face and neck and gently massage in with a water-in-oil cream. Leave for 15 minutes before tissuing off.
- Apply unrefined vegetable oil under the eyes and pat in (don't rub).
- Apply make-up.

P.M.

- Remove make-up with unrefined vegetable oil or a suitable water-in-oil cleanser. Apply and wait for one minute before removing with a wet and warm, but not hot, face flannel. Repeat several times until all traces of make-up have gone.
- Apply milk or a suitable oil-in-water emulsion and remove with moistened cotton wool. Repeat.
- Wash and rinse as above. Apply freshener.
- Mix water-in-oil cream and petroleum jelly (half and half) in the palm of the hand and apply to face and neck.
- Apply unrefined vegetable oil under the eyes and pat in.

## Additional Treatments

- Exfoliate with oatmeal twice a week (see page 99).
- Practise facial exercises a minimum of three times a week (see page 82).
- Apply Anti-Wrinkle and Antioxidant Cream Skin Food (see page 97) to face and neck at least twice a week in addition to normal moisturizing (see page 89).
- Apply the Three in One Skin Care Treatment (see page 99) twice a week.

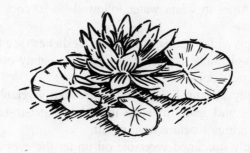

*Part Five*

# Some More Recipes

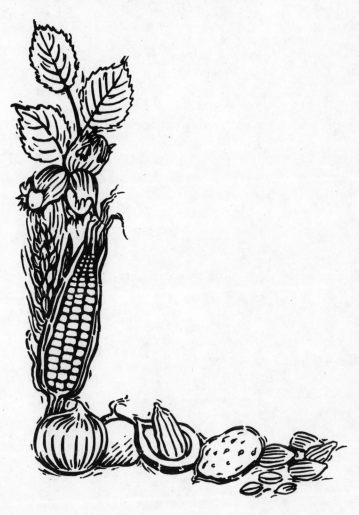

# Cereals

## Crunchy Fruit Munch

*Serves 2*

150g (5oz/1 cup) pecans, chopped
½ apple, unpeeled, cored and diced
½ banana, sliced
½ pear, unpeeled, cored and diced
70g (2¾oz/½ cup) raisins
4 figs, chopped
2 tablespoons wheatgerm

Combine all the ingredients. Add milk or plain yogurt.

## Nut and Seed Cereal

*Serves 2*

50g (2oz/½ cup) wheatgerm
60g (2½oz/½ cup) sunflower seeds, ground
65g (2½oz/½ cup) sesame seeds
25g (1oz/¼ cup) walnuts, chopped
40g (1½oz/¼ cup) rice polishings or brown rice, cooked

Combine all the ingredients. Add milk or plain yogurt and serve.

## Enzyme-packed Cereal

*Serves 1–2*

4 tablespoons fresh wheatgerm
3 teaspoons sunflower seeds
3 teaspoons sesame seeds
2 teaspoons rice polishings or brown rice, cooked
4 teaspoons brewers' yeast
150g (5oz/1 cup) fresh fruit, chopped

Combine all the ingredients and serve with whole milk or freshly squeezed orange juice.

## High-energy Muesli

Serves 12

450g (1lb) rolled oats, crushed
100g (4oz) sunflower seeds
100g (4oz) wheatgerm
50g (2oz) almonds, unblanched and
    ground
50g (2oz) hazelnuts, ground
50g (2oz) Brazil nuts, ground
100g (4oz) raisins, washed
40g (1½oz/½ cup) dates, stoned and
    chopped
40g (1½oz/½ cup) dried apricots*,
    chopped
1 banana, sliced
honey to taste (optional)
plain yogurt

Combine all the ingredients, except the banana, honey and yogurt and store in an air-tight jar in the refrigerator. Add the banana, honey and yogurt to each portion when serving.

## Swiss Breakfast

Serves 2

2 apples, unpeeled, cored and grated
150g (5oz/1 cup) fresh berries or
    grapes, peaches or bananas, sliced
25g (1oz/¼ cup) juice of 1 lemon
25g (1oz/¼ cup) nuts, chopped
150ml (5 fl oz) plain yogurt
75g (3oz/½ cup) raw oats
    (oatmeal), soaked overnight in
    300ml (10 fl oz) of water
2 tablespoons fresh wheatgerm

Combine all the ingredients. Serve with freshly squeezed orange juice.

* Use sun-dried not sulphur-dried fruit.

## Thermos-cooked Cereal

40g (1½oz/¼ cup) whole barley
40g (1½oz/¼ cup) whole rye
225g (8oz/¼ cup) brown rice
25g (1oz/⅛ cup) whole millet
25g (1oz/¼ cup) wheatgerm
25g (1oz/¼ cup) sunflower seeds

*Serves 5*

Blend all the ingredients. Take 165g (5½oz/½ cup) of this cereal mixture, sufficient for 2 servings and stir it into 300ml (½pt/2 cups) of boiling water. Allow to simmer for 2 minutes and then pour the contents into a wide-necked Thermos flask. Replace cap and lay the Thermos on its side. Wake up the following morning to a hot cereal ready to be served with either milk or yogurt and honey. (Store any unused, uncooked cereal in an airtight container.)

# Side Salads

## Cabbage and Watercress Salad

225g (8oz/2 cups) white cabbage,
    shredded
25g (1oz/1 cup) watercress
2 tablespoons sultanas
1 tablespoon finely chopped onion
salad dressing of your choice (see
    pages 179–81)
freshly ground black pepper to taste

*Serves 2*

Toss all the ingredients in a bowl, add the pepper, mix thoroughly and serve.

## Celery and Pineapple Salad

225g (8oz/2 cups) celery, chopped
225g (8oz/2 cups) fresh pineapple,
    cut into chunks
salad dressing of your choice (see
    pages 179–81)

*Serves 2–3*

Toss all the ingredients in a bowl, mix thoroughly and serve.

## Raw Pea Salad

Serves 2–3

175g (6oz/1 cup) fresh, raw peas
300g (72oz/2 cups) carrot, grated
150g (6oz/1 cup) sunflower seeds
1 small onion, chopped
salad dressing of your choice (see
    pages 179–81)

Toss all the ingredients together in a bowl, mix thoroughly and serve.

## Fruity Winter Salad

Serves 2–3

175g (6oz/1 cup) apples, finely
    chopped
100g (4oz/1 cup) celery, finely
    chopped
100g (4oz/1 cup) cabbage, finely
    chopped
15g (½oz/½ cup) watercress,
    chopped
4 tablespoons freshly squeezed
    orange juice
lettuce, pieces

Toss all the ingredients, except the lettuce, in the orange juice and leave to marinate for a few hours. Serve on the bed of lettuce.

## Carrot and Raisin Salad Supreme

Serves 2

250g (9oz/1½ cups) carrots, grated
65g (2½oz/½ cup) raisins
65ml (2½ fl oz/¼ cup) freshly
    squeezed lemon juice
mayonnaise to taste
25g (1oz) lettuce

Soak the raisins in the lemon juice overnight, until they are plump. Combine them with the carrots and sufficient mayonnaise to moisten. Serve on a bed of lettuce.

## Winter Salad Surprise

*Serves 2–3*

*100g (4oz/1 cup) cabbage, finely*
*   shredded*
*175g (6oz/1 cup) carrots, grated*
*100g (4oz/1 cup) celery, finely*
*   chopped*
*100g (4oz/1 cup) red pepper,*
*   chopped*
*4 tablespoons French dressing*
*300ml (10 fl oz/1 cup) unsweetened*
*   pineapple juice*
*lettuce, pieces or watercress*

Toss the vegetables in the dressing and
combine with the pineapple juice. Serve
on a bed of lettuce or watercress.

## Nut Salad Special

*Serves 3–4*

*150g (5oz/1 cup) pecans, chopped*
*150g (5oz/1 cup) walnuts, chopped*
*100g (4oz/1 cup) apple, unpeeled,*
*   cored and sliced*
*25g (1oz/1 cup) lettuce, shredded*
*8 dates, stoned and chopped*
*20g (¾oz/¼ cup) fresh coconut,*
*   shredded*
*3 tablespoons raisins*
*French dressing to taste*

Combine all the ingredients. Toss in the
French dressing and serve.

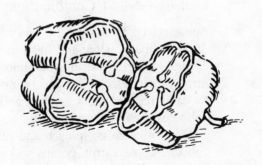

## Salad Richmond

*Serves 2–3*

50g (2oz/1 cup) mung beansprouts
50g (2oz/1 cup) sprouted wheat
65g (2½oz/½ cup) sunflower seeds
65g (2½oz/½ cup) onion, chopped
150g (5oz/½ cup) avocado, peeled,
   stoned and diced
15g (½oz/½ cup) watercress,
   chopped
salad dressing of your choice (see
   pages 179–81)

Combine the sprouts, seeds, onion, avocado and watercress. Toss in the dressing and serve.

## Protein Salad

*Serves 2–3*

50g (2oz/1 cup) sprouted wheat
25g (1oz/½ cup) mung beansprouts
100g (4oz/½ cup) sprouted chickpeas
100g (4oz/1 cup) red pepper,
   chopped
65g (2½oz/½ cup) onion, diced
fresh parsley, chopped, to taste
French dressing to taste

Combine the sprouts, red pepper and onion. Toss in the French dressing. Sprinkle with parsley and serve.

## Delicious Salad Combinations

Apple, celery, raisins, pecans and banana
Apple, cabbage, celery and fresh mint
Apple, watercress, raisins and almonds
Apple, watercress, radish and pumpkin seeds
Avocado, red pepper, watercress and sunflower seeds
Cabbage, watercress and raisins
Cabbage, watercress, spinach and garlic
Cabbage, apple, carrot, pecans and sunflower seeds
Carrot, apple and raisins
Carrot, apple, celery, radish, red cabbage, parsley, raisins, apricots
   and almonds

Carrot, beet, lettuce, alfalfa sprouts and avocado
Carrot, red pepper, celery and parsley
Carrot, celery, watercress, and mixed nuts
Carrot and fresh pineapple
Celery, apple, figs and dates
Chicory, endive, watercress and onion
Cucumber, tomato, green peas and onion
Cucumber, tomato, avocado and sunflower seeds
Endive, tomato and watercress
Endive, orange and watercress
Green beans (steamed), onion, celery, pepper and walnuts
Lettuce, endive, chicory, watercress and onion
Lettuce, apple, radish, onion, dates, raisins, walnuts and sesame
    seeds
Lettuce, alfalfa sprouts, mung beansprouts, sesame seeds, and garlic
Lettuce, celery, alfalfa sprouts, pumpkin and sunflower seeds
Mung beansprouts, celery, caraway seeds and pecans
Spinach (raw), apple, mung beansprouts and onion
Tomato, green pepper, parsley, avocado and onion
Watercress, avocado, cabbage and pumpkin seeds

# Salad Dressings

## Honey Dressing

2 tablespoons honey
85ml (3 fl oz/½ cup) apple cider
    vinegar
¼ teaspoon freshly ground black
    pepper
¼ teaspoon mustard powder
1 teaspoon sea salt (optional)
300ml (10 fl oz/1 cup) vegetable oil,
    cold-pressed

Combine all the ingredients except the oil.
Then, add the oil a little at a time until
the mixture is well blended.
This dressing is delicious with a green
salad.

## Avocado Dressing

1 ripe avocado, peeled, stoned and
   mashed
300ml (10 fl oz/1 cup) plain yogurt
1 tablespoon soy sauce
pinch of oregano

Blend all the ingredients until smooth.
Serve over brussels sprouts or a green
salad.
This is a favourite dressing of mine for it
is smooth, and tastes delicious and rather
luxurious.

## Fruit Delight

1 ripe avocado, peeled, stoned and
   mashed
1 large grapefruit, peeled and
   segmented
1 large tomato, skinned and chopped

Place all the ingredients in a liquidizer
and blend until smooth.
This dressing can be added to vegetable
salads or simply used as a dip.

## Simple French Dressing

500ml (17 fl oz/¾ cup) vegetable
   oil, cold-pressed
65ml (2½ fl oz/¼ cup) freshly
   squeezed lemon juice
2 teaspoons honey
1 clove garlic, crushed

Place all the ingredients in a jar with a
screw-type lid and shake well.

## Herb Dressing

1 clove garlic, crushed
¼ teaspoon anise seeds, ground
¼ teaspoon mixed herbs, ground
¼ teaspoon dill, ground
¼ teaspoon mint, ground
¼ teaspoon tarragon, ground
85ml (3 fl oz/1½ cup) olive oil,
   cold-pressed
75ml (6 fl oz/⅔ cup) freshly
   squeezed lemon juice

Mix the garlic and anise seeds. Add the
garlic mixture and all the herbs to the oil
and the lemon juice. Pour into a bottle
and refrigerate. Shake well before use.

## Sunshine Salad Dressing

65ml (2½ fl oz/¼ cup) sunflower
oil, cold-pressed
65ml (2½ fl oz/¼ cup) olive oil,
cold-pressed
65ml (2½ fl oz/¼ cup) peanut oil,
cold-pressed
65ml (2½ fl oz/¼ cup) freshly
squeezed lemon juice
½ tablespoon wheatgerm oil, cold-
pressed
1 teaspoon honey
½ clove garlic, crushed

Place all the ingredients in a jar with a
screw-lid and shake well.
This dressing is suitable for any kind of
salad.

## Buttermilk Dressing

65ml (2½ fl oz/¼ cup) buttermilk
30g (2oz/¼ cup) plain, low-fat
cottage cheese
1 teaspoon finely chopped onion
½ small clove garlic, crushed
1 teaspoon chopped fresh dill or
¼ teaspoon dried dill

Combine the ingredients and pour over
lettuce or any green salad.

## Yogurt and Dill Dressing

150ml (5 fl oz/½ cup) plain yogurt
1½ teaspoons chopped fresh dill or
½ teaspoon dried dill
½ spring onion, finely chopped

Combine the ingredients and pour over
any type of salad – it is particularly good
with cucumber.

# Desserts

## Hawaii Delight

Serves 3

½ fresh, ripe pineapple, peeled, cored
and finely chopped
40g (1½oz/½ cup) fresh coconut,
shredded, unsweetened
1½ tablespoons honey

Combine all the ingredients and serve.

## Apricot Crème

Serves 3

225g (8oz/½ lb) dried apricots,
unsulphured
300ml (10 fl oz/1 cup) plain yogurt
honey to taste

Place the apricots in a bowl, cover with water and leave to soak overnight. The following day, put the apricots and the liquid in which they were soaked in a liquidizer and blend until smooth. Stir in the yogurt and honey and serve.

## Fruit Yogurt Sundae

Serves 2

1 apple, cored and quartered
1 banana, cut lengthwise and in half
25g (1oz/¼ cup) wheatgerm
300ml (10 fl oz/1 cup) plain yogurt
25g (1oz/¼ cup) mixed nuts and
seeds, chopped

Place the apple with a dash of water in a liquidizer and blend until smooth. Spoon the puree equally into two sundae dishes. Top with the banana pieces and sprinkle with wheatgerm. Add the yogurt and sprinkle with the mixed nuts and seeds.

## Nutty Pineapple Dessert

Serves 3

½ large, ripe pineapple, peeled, cored
and sliced
150g (5 oz/1 cup) almonds, finely
grated
250g (9oz/¾ cup) honey

Place a layer of pineapple in a bowl and sprinkle with some of the nuts and honey. Add another layer of pineapple, nuts and honey and continue until all the ingredients are used. Chill for 2 hours before serving.

## Berry Yogurt

**Serves 2**

450g (1 lb/3 cups) strawberries or
  raspberries or *any seasonal
  berries*
300ml (10 fl oz/1 cup) plain yogurt
75g (3oz/ ¼ cup) honey

Pour 25g (1oz/ ¼ cup) of the berries, the yogurt and the honey into a liquidizer and blend until smooth. Spoon it over the remaining berries and serve.

# Spreads

## Peanut Butter

150g (5 oz/1 cup) raw peanuts
1–2 teaspoons vegetable oil, cold-
  pressed
pinch sea salt (optional)

Pour all the ingredients into a liquidizer and blend until either crunchy or smooth according to taste.

## Nutty Date Spread

175g (6oz/1 cup) dates, stoned
150ml (5 fl oz/2 cup) mixed nuts
1 small carton plain yogurt

Place the dates and the nuts in a liquidizer, add 3 tablespoons of yogurt and blend until smooth. Add more yogurt sufficient to make a spreadable paste. It is delicious either as a spread or as a topping for salads or fresh fruit desserts.

## Hummus

2 tablespoons freshly squeezed lemon
  juice
5 tablespoons sesame oil, cold-
  pressed
1 large clove garlic
450g (1 lb/16oz) cooked chickpeas
freshly ground black pepper to taste

Place all the ingredients in a liquidizer, blend until smooth, and serve.

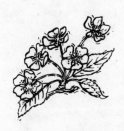

## Nut and Seed Butter

275g (10oz/2 cups) mixed unsalted
    nuts (cashews, pecans, walnuts
    and almonds are good)
150g (5oz/1 cup) sunflower seeds
    shelled
150g (5oz/1 cup) sesame seeds
oil, cold-pressed, to blend
honey to taste

Place the nuts and seeds in a liquidizer,
add the oil, a little at a time and blend
until you have a spreadable paste. Mix in
the honey and serve.

## Chicken Liver Pâté

100g (4oz) chicken livers
25g (1oz) onion, finely sliced
2 tablespoons chicken stock or water
freshly ground black pepper to taste
pinch of thyme
pinch of marjoram
50g (2oz) cottage cheese
1 teaspoon tomato purée
1 teaspoon Worcestershire sauce

Poach the chicken livers with the onion,
stock or water, seasoning and herbs, in a
covered pan over a low heat for about 10
minutes. Pour the mixture into a
liquidizer. Add the cottage cheese, tomato
purée and Worcestershire sauce and blend
until smooth. Serve.

## Smoked Mackerel Pâté

50g (2oz) smoked mackerel fillet
2 teaspoons finely chopped onion
2 teaspoons freshly squeezed lemon
    juice
10g (1¼oz) mock butter (see page
    75)
freshly ground black pepper to taste

Place all the ingredients in a liquidizer
and blend until smooth. Serve.

# Health Drinks

## Molasses Milk Shake

Serves 2

600ml (1 pint) skimmed milk
2 tablespoons low-fat powdered milk
2 teaspoons unsulphured molasses

Place all the ingredients in a liquidizer and blend until smooth. Refrigerate. Shake before serving.

## Orange Milk Shake

Serves 2

2 glasses freshly squeezed orange juice
4 tablespoons low-fat powdered milk
2 tablespoons honey

Place all the ingredients in a liquidizer and blend until smooth. Serve.

## Complexion Cocktail for Dry Skin

Serves 1

300ml (10 fl oz/1 cup) freshly
  squeezed orange juice
1 egg yolk
2 teaspoons peanut oil, unrefined
1 tablespoon wheatgerm
1 teaspoon honey

Place all the ingredients in a liquidizer and blend until smooth. Serve.

## Banana Milk Shake

Serves 1–2

600ml (1pt/3 cups) skimmed milk
1 tablespoon low-fat powdered milk
1 large, ripe banana
1 tablespoon honey (optional)

Place all the ingredients in a liquidizer and blend until smooth. Serve.

## Nutty Carrot Cocktail

Serves 2

150ml (5 fl oz/½ cup) freshly
   prepared carrot juice
150ml (5 fl oz/½ cup) skimmed milk
25g (1oz/¼ cup) blanched almonds,
   chopped
3 teaspoons wheatgerm

Place all the ingredients in a liquidizer
and blend until smooth. Serve.

## Protein Health Drink

Serves 2–3

40g (1½oz/¼ cup) sunflower seeds
25g (1oz/¼ cup) blanched almonds
900ml (1½pt/3 cups) cold water
1 teaspoon low-fat powdered milk
2 tablespoons honey

Place the sunflower seeds, almonds and
one cup (300ml, 10 fl oz) of the water in
a liquidizer and leave to soak for 15
minutes. Then, blend until smooth. Add
the remaining ingredients, including the
water, and blend until smooth.

## Casis Milk

Serves 2

600ml (1pt/2 cups) skimmed milk
6 dates, chopped
2 tablespoons coconut, shredded
3 teaspoons wheatgerm
2 teaspoons safflower oil, cold-pressed

Place all the ingredients in a liquidizer
and blend until smooth. Serve.

## Vegetable Fruit Punch

Serves 2

150ml (5 fl oz/½ cup) freshly
   prepared carrot juice
150ml (5 fl oz/½ cup freshly
   prepared papaya juice
1 banana
3 dates, chopped
2 tablespoons wheatgerm

Place all the ingredients in a liquidizer
and blend until smooth. Serve.

186

## Tomato Punch

Serves 2

300ml (10 fl oz/2 cups) freshly
   squeezed tomato juice
2 teaspoons chopped fresh parsley
2 teaspoons freshly squeezed lemon
   juice
4 teaspoons brewers' yeast

Place all the ingredients in a liquidizer
and blend until smooth. Serve.

## Apple Grape Glory

Serves 2

300ml (10 fl oz/1 cup) freshly
   prepared apple juice
150ml (5 fl oz/½ cup) freshly
   prepared grape juice
65g (2½oz/¼ cup) raisins
2 teaspoons plain yogurt
2 teaspoons brewers' yeast

Place all the ingredients in a liquidizer
and blend until smooth. Serve.

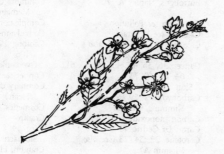

# Index